You Can't Quit Until You Know What's Eating You

Overcoming Compulsive Eating

Donna LeBlanc, M.Ed., L.P.C.

Health Communications, Inc.
Deerfield Beach, Florida

Library of Congress Cataloging-in-Publication Data

LeBlanc, Donna
    You can't quit until you know what's eating you: overcoming compulsive eating / Donna LeBlanc.
        p.   cm.
    ISBN 1-55874-103-8: $7.95
    1. Compulsive eating.   2. Obesity — Psychological aspects. I. Title.
    RC552.C65L33   1990   90-4761
    616.85'26—dc20   CIP

ISBN 1-55874-103-8

Publisher: Health Communications, Inc.
            3201 S.W. 15th Street
            Deerfield Beach, Florida 33442-8124

Cover design by Graphic Expressions

DEDICATION

To Galadriel Mohan for her brilliance
in polishing this work.

To those who suffer in silence from the
problem of compulsive eating. There is hope.

To Bill DeFoore for his encouragement
and assistance in putting my work into print.
I am deeply grateful. Thank you.

CONTENTS

Introduction

It was only a room away—fragrant, moist and rich.

The more she thought she shouldn't touch it—she ought to wait for Bob and Mickie, etc.—the more optimistic she felt about tomorrow. Tomorrow she would stop eating the fattening fun stuff. Tomorrow self-control would, or could, be easier. Any day would be easier than today, easier than right now.

NOW, she was going to eat it because she wanted it and it was there and whatever else she needed in her life wasn't.

She ate it.

A lot of it.

In fact, all of it.

It was the sixth day after the final day of her third dieting program this year. Like World War II, the last diet was supposed to be the one that was to end all wars. But that wasn't what was happening. The conflict wore on, half of her begging for the joy of sugar and half pretending that an eternity of self-denial was a realistic goal.

This book is for people who are tired of failure and its negative effect on both their self-esteem and their bodies.

It is for those who find diets an exercise in futility, who are tired of hiding their appetites from others and who are ready to get rid of guilt and self-blame for good.

It offers a way out for the 300 pound overweight and for the five pound overweight—the common denominator of these two being a loss of control over achieving their favorite reading on the scales.

What Block Blocks Permanent Loss?

As I have seen in my own history of compulsive eating, mechanical or format solutions seldom last. However, not everyone who wants to shed pounds is ready to shed what is at the crux of permanent weight loss: the fear of examining those feelings that have been causing us psychological indigestion for many years.

In our quest for the real triggers of our urges to over-eat, we will visit the dining rooms, kitchens and eating "hideouts" of a number of people with the same concerns. We will hear from many I've seen in my practice as a specialist in eating disorders. As we listen to their experiences, we'll understand better that the agonies that foster compulsive eating can be faced and shared without shame or blame. Their stories will be altered just enough to ensure anonymity.

We also will take a look at old notions of what we need to survive and will re-examine the models we've accepted and the standards we have set for ourselves. Are they really ours or someone else's? When is abandoning "will-power" a virtue, not a vice?

The entire issue of will power versus doing what we feel like doing is central to defeating permanent weight loss. Setting up an internal battleground between the Forces of Fat and the Admirable Abstainer is a common *modus operandi* among compulsive eaters who cycle in and out of diets. It results in heady short-term victories with some people, during which they feel very good about themselves as victors. Then come the dismal regressions during which the sense of defeat and failure often oozes inappropriately throughout other areas of self-regard.

The Strife-Free Approach

A true understanding of what's eating us—of what really is behind the reason food is so important in our lives—eliminates the need for "artificial" discipline and conflict. Our Inner Child and our Critical Parent stop their wrangling and allow our Adult self to flower fully, to get on with the satisfactions of life, free from the tyranny of emotionally driven appetites.

We can learn to stop sabotaging our attempts at permanent weight loss if the determination for compassionate understanding of ourselves is there. After I started the Compulsive Eating Program—based on my experience as a staff psychologist with major weight-loss program—I saw the power of real insight to change lives impressively. Becoming healthier and happier, people experience the joy of being at home in their bodies, proud of who they are and what they have achieved. As they work through their emotional blocks, using various exercises developed to make insights come more easily, their excess weight begins to disappear.

All this takes place without conscious dieting.

While insights are vital to weighing what we want to weigh, they seldom can stand alone. They need repeating, restating, underlining and highlighting—just as we've done throughout the years with the misleading negative affirmations that have kept us too heavy.

Exercising Your Insight

The power of the past cannot be dismissed lightly in the excitement of vital new understanding. So throughout the book, you will find affirmations and visualization exercises which can be practiced daily to strengthen your new "muscles" of insight. These are valuable aids in the process of reprogramming our conditioned minds and of permanently shaking up the patterns that we've followed helplessly for too long.

You'll find these exercises throughout the book, wherever they may be helpful. It's a good idea to take advantage of them at the point where they occur before going on to new material. They will reinforce the discovery process and make it possible for you to identify even more profoundly with others. You may very well find, as a result, that the foundation of someone else's eating disorder may be startlingly similar to yours, even though you've considered your circumstances either irrelevant to your eating or a unique personal situation.

Our elation over seeing that it is possible, at last, to claim our right to a more satisfying life will be our motivation for practicing these reinforcers.

The payoff? Curbed urges to eat compulsively, a slimmer, fitter body and a raised level of self-esteem.

How slim, you say? We all have the power within to be as slim as we want but—sometimes—we may want to rest from the activity of renewal before we go on. After all, changing the mind and body patterns of years takes a little more effort than swallowing a mint truffle. After some exploratory weight loss, we may find that a considerably lowered level of weight is so pleasant that we're happy to rest there and enjoy it for a while. We might even entertain the idea that, at a certain point, some extra weight is either okay or okay for a while—if we are able to make this weight level genuinely our choice, not an echo from a misunderstood past.

Not Every "Thin One" Wants Out

It's not always true, as critic-writer Cyril Connolly expressed it, that "Inside every fat man, a thin one is wildly signaling to be let out." To the contrary, once in therapy, many are wildly signaling to be left in, safely insulated from facing a host of difficulties, mostly interpersonal. Yet the pressures to be healthier, to be thinner, come from so many directions—advertising, the workplace, family, friends, our doctors. There are so many of these demands that pressure itself may become the issue ("Nobody's going to tell me how I should be!"), clouding the underlying cause.

Frankly, fat has become the best friend of many. "Not me!" you say. "No way. It's disgusting, I hate it. I've spent half my life trying to lose it and I've been on every diet there is. Even the 120-Day Norwegian Tundra-and-Stork-Steak Diet. And I've got a ten-speed exercycle, and . . . "

That may well be true for you but the best spirit in which to begin this book is one of all-out openness in the exploration of what makes us eat compulsively. Feel free to experiment with yourself, your feelings and your early food memories in the safety zone of this no-fault approach to permanent weight reduction.

Dare To Know Yourself

Test drive feelings you might ordinarily reject out-of-hand. There's no obligation. Finding out if, deep down, we really don't want to lose weight may rank first on our agenda. We need to gently poke our inner selves to release valuable information. Does part of us need, on some level, to stay fat? For many people there is a fear of losing the relationship with food they've built over many years because of what it has really meant in their lives. Food has been their best friend and fat, their protection—facts that didn't make sense and therefore were buried deep down. Everyone knows food and fat are your enemies! This is a confusing message.

So, before we begin one of the most interesting and rewarding trips we will ever take—a journey with plenty of companions around the world of compulsive eating—

we should define our own perspective on food. How do
we conduct our extra eating?

- Do we eat a lot all day? Are our bodies obese?
- Are we secret eaters—nobody really knows how we
  manage to gain?
- Are we not fat at all or only slightly overweight but
  what we do eat is bad for us?
- No matter how many times we try to reform our
  diet, do we find that we invariably reject good food in
  favor of junk?
- Have we been stuck for too long in the scary states of
  borderline or full-fledged bulimia or anorexia— hy-
  percompulsive eating and its opposite, hypercompul-
  sive food avoidance? (More about these special problems later.)

A Most Natural Way To Lose It

A lot of questions lie between us and gaining control
over ourselves.

As we see what we're made of psychologically, the
straight answers will come to us and the pounds will go,
without dieting, without starvation. You will be losing
weight naturally, nurturing the inner you without overeating. You will be able to express anger, not smother it in
whipped cream.

You will no longer be locked into a set of behaviors
that you are unable to change—patterns of thought, actions and feelings that all lead to extra servings, odd-
hour nibbling.

The compulsive eating cycle will have been broken at
last. You will have a new shape but it won't feel strange.
It will seem like remodeling your body to feel more like
the home you have always deserved.

Understanding Compulsive Eating

Sixty to 70 million people in the United States are compulsive eaters, according to one conservative estimate. (The very, very few with an actual physiological basis for excess weight aren't included in this count.)

How do you know if you're among them? Not everyone who is overweight wants to be associated with the term "compulsive." But remember, it describes a person's conditioning, not character. Here's an informal guide that will help you evaluate your relationship to some of the major factors behind chronic overweight.

Compulsive Eating Questionnaire

What Control Do You Really Have Over Your Eating?

1. **How often do you find yourself eating something you wish you hadn't?**

    a. Sometimes b. Frequently c. Daily
    d. More than once a day

2. **How long has this been happening?**
    a. Six months to a year b. One to two years
    c. More than two years d. Since childhood

3. **When do you believe was the first time you started eating compulsively?**
    a. This past year b. A few years ago
    c. Many years ago d. As a child

4. **How overweight would you say you are?**
    a. Five to 10 pounds b. 11 to 25 c. 26 to 50
    d. More

5. **How long have you been going on diets to lose?**
    a. Six months to a year b. One to five years
    c. More than five d. Since childhood

6. **How did you, personally, find the atmosphere in your home as a child?**
    a. Happy, peaceful b. Tense c. Lonely
    d. Scary, threatening

7. **To what degree was food used in your childhood home as a sign of love, a reward for good behavior, a punishment or a friend to fill lonely hours?**
    a. Hardly ever b. Sometimes c. Often d. Daily

8. **Over the past 10 years, has your problem with food increased?**
    Yes   No

9. **Was there any drug or alcohol abuse by your parents?**
    Yes   No

10. **Did either parent ever have a problem with weight?**
    Yes   No

11. **Have you ever been afraid of being attractive or wanted to hide your body?**
    a. Hardly ever b. Sometimes c. Frequently
    d. Always

12. **Besides eating for enjoyment, do you use food for comfort or for something to do?**
    a. Hardly ever b. Sometimes c. Often d. Daily

13. **Do you often eat secretly?**
    Yes   No
14. **Do you regard food as "the enemy?"**
    a. Hardly ever   b. Sometimes   c. Frequently
    d. Always

Scoring: Total one point for every (a) answer, two points for every (b) answer, three points for (c) answers and four points for (d) answers. A "no" gets one point, a "yes," two.
10 to 15 points: "Fun food" may be even more important to you than you think. It would be easiest on you and your body if you could take charge now.
16-21 points: Both your mind and body are becoming used to extra pounds. It's time to look beyond diets to a permanent solution.
22-29 points: Although you rarely can say *no* to the temptation of food, you don't have to continue fighting it. Gaining a better understanding of yourself will prove to be your most effective weight-loss program.
30-40 or more points: Fat thinks it's found a permanent home but you haven't given up. Hurray! Despite what has become a chronic condition—reinforced by a lot of psychological conditioning—you still believe in change. As you learn reasons to believe in yourself, you'll watch those numbers on the scales drop.

Compulsive Eating: Losing Control

You don't have to be just one of the estimated 34 million who are "officially" overweight, which is defined as 20 percent more than ideal body weight.

You don't have to be 200, 100, 50 or even just five pounds overweight to qualify as having lost control over your eating (that's the basic definition of compulsive eating).

Compulsive eaters are people who continue to eat when they should stop, who go ahead and eat something they wish they had turned down.

(Feeling squeamish and embarrassed as you read this? Guilt is one of the many indicators that compulsive eating has you in its grip.)

Compulsive eaters don't give in just once in a while. Giving in has become a way of life, a way of coping.

Note the "has become." Extra weight or food guilt wasn't always part of who they were. In the Compulsive Eating, where we're after permanent results, we re-establish contact with our bedrock natures that have been covered up by negative coping techniques such as compulsive eating. For many of us, these techniques reach back into early childhood.

The Extremes And The Mid-Pointers

The nth degree of compulsive eating is bulimia. The word comes to us from the Greek for "ox" *(bous)* and "hunger" *(limos)* and it refers to a continous, abnormal appetite ("hungry as an ox"). Bulimia is eating in a binge/purge fashion, gorging and throwing up, although the latter usual result is not always part of the condition. It differs from compulsive eating because of the amounts of food eaten, not the weight gained.

Garden variety compulsive eating can include binging: eating industrial-size quantities of food in a short period. Once the compulsive eating urge flares up, a sense of additional haste to meet the needy feeling takes over. The thought process may be: "This is special and I may never get this chance again . . ." or "This has been held back from me for so long . . ."

A single-minded desperation sets in. We turn into animals, although mostly the friendly, tail-wagging variety. Ravenous, we now know what makes Fido tick. We gotta get to that bowl, and fast. Gulp, gulp, gulp and it's gone. Not until the container, plate or bag is empty do we come to our senses. "What have I done (again)?!" We feel like Jack-the-Ripper-of-Junk-Foods.

The opposite extreme is anorexia (*an-*, without; *orexis*, a desire for). People with anorexia can actually starve themselves to death. Many are terrified that they are on the verge of becoming obese even though the mirror reflects a figure that, to everyone else, looks emaciated.

In between are those who struggle with an appetite less radically manifested. Perhaps you specialize in items you know are bad for you. Maybe you just can't seem to stop when you've started on certain foods; you have lost your eating "brakes." Once into a pie, you're committed until the end of the "relationship," which is a lot sooner than you had planned at the time of purchase. Yours may not be the type of eating that schedules four bagels and three bags of junk food daily. But perhaps you've come to feel that a meal without dessert is like a day without sunshine.

Should finding a description of your habits here make you feel very uneasy, alarmed or panicky, that's natural and healthy. Let yourself feel it. It's a process between The Urgent Urge and gratification that we routinely skip when caught up in the cycle of compulsive eating.

Not Me

In lieu of panic when we once again feel ourselves capitulating to compulsive eating, we substitute denial — one of the ways we manage to live with our imperfections. When we're face-to-face with the facts, we often want to duck.

Realizing you're a compulsive eater, however, is not the same as being charged with a felony. It is not a crime against personhood. It is very human and therefore very common, as the statistics show. You can approach it as you would any other habit, making the decision to live with it or live without it.

Like other habits, it is acquired, not hard-wired into our lives. It does serve the quasi-positive function of reducing stress over an issue or issues we don't know how to face otherwise. It is only when it creates yet another

problem of great concern to us that we become motivated
to dump it for good.

Games Compulsive Eaters Play

Some of us who are obviously overweight and constantly talking to our friends about diets and calories still
don't hesitate to deny that we're eating too much. We've
cut out this and that and that and this and STILL weight
comes out of nowhere and attaches itself to us. Maybe,
like radon, it's seeping up through the kitchen floor?

Kerry was a longtime member of a well-known weight-
loss program—a woman in her mid-40s with an otherwise
engagingly frank personality—who insisted, with the
most innocent of baby blue eyes, that she retained so
much weight because "I just can't stay away from fruit!
Especially cherries!"

Cherry cordials, you say? No, the little raw reds, she
insists. Well, maybe, if you're a binging fruit bat, but human metabolism needs more than fruit to slow it down. It
could be that Kerry fixed on fruit as a delicate overindul-
gence and not as much associated with failure as walnut
cheese tortes and sausage, her true loves.

Ned was a clinical instructor at a local university, inclined to gentle banter at parties—except at the party
where we started talking about compulsive eating. He
brought it up and, because he was overweight, I thought
he was talking about a subject that concerned him personally. Not so, he insisted.

"What do you eat sort of compulsively?" I asked genially,
after exposing my current favorite junk foods.

"Oh, but I don't," he snapped, his eyebrows arched in
warning. "I just don't get any exercise."

Despite the eyebrows and because we were friends, I
pursued the source of his still unaccounted for extra
weight. It seemed that he connected the term compulsive
eating with "neurotic" behavior—which he didn't associ-

ate with himself. He did, however, work very long hours and when he put in a tiring day he would come home and extra-eat—a carton of chocolate chip mint ice cream, alternating with nonfat (but sugary) frozen yogurt—potato chips with a dip of sour cream and chives.

But in his mind, this wasn't compulsive eating; it was "a little treat. My way of being good to myself. I deserve something nice for days like that!"

When I asked him how he would feel if he came home to a treat that wasn't edible or to a non-fat, no-sugar, no-honey, etc. snack, he just looked at me blankly. "Doesn't sound like much to look forward to," he said finally.

Another form of denial is particularly sad because it separates some of us from the normal enjoyment of sharing special meals with friends. Aileen, a social services caseworker with a wide circle of friends at her office, is frequently asked to go out to lunch with co-workers, but complained to me that she dreads these occasions and avoids many of them.

"I love food, not just fattening things, but I always feel compelled to have a salad when I'm with other people. I'm sorry, I know how good they are for you and I like them occasionally, but the last thing I want at lunch is a salad. I want something hearty—and a dessert—for my midday meal. But in front of all these people who are forever talking about dieting, I feel I've got to show some self-control. I try to convince myself that it's a good opportunity to eat something I need but, basically, I wish I could go and eat somewhere by myself."

Food Rhymes With Mood

There's a good reason why we don't reach for "good" foods when we want to reward ourselves or escape from a frustrating day. The good stuff does not give us immediate gratification and we're not looking just for nourishment. Physiologists have shown us that we are drawn to certain foods at certain times because they have unusual properties either to stimulate or pacify. The top two foods in this category are sugar and chocolate.

Volumes have been written about what sugar does to our brains. The ups and downs it creates are notorious.

Research studies on chocolate have revealed that it prompts a chemical change in the blood that is identical to the chemistry of someone in love. Have you ever noticed how sensuous the chocolate commercials are? Generally, they present a situation in which an individual is obsessed or having a love affair with chocolate. Chocolate is so potent that the term "chocoholic" is readily understood by anyone whose tastes run in this direction.

Any food can become psychologically addictive as we cross the line between enjoying something occasionally and setting up an automatic expectation for it by our bodies as well as our minds. Ten o'clock comes and where are our raised glazed doughnuts? The stomach rumbles, the mind grumbles. We look forward to them every weekday and today the doughnut shop is sold out? World-class depression sets in.

Restyle your appetite, say some weight loss programs. Train yourself to binge on carrot sticks instead.

How long would that last? For most of us, long enough not to want to see anything long and orange ever again. You might be pressured into an alternative similar to that indulged in by many who decide to eat only healthy foods. They eat large quantities of healthy foods—say, a box of fruit-sweetened whole-wheat carob chip cookies a day. No saturated fats, no preservatives, no chocolate, no weight loss.

The need that we are trying to fill cannot be met by carrot sticks or carrot cake. Edibles, no matter how many or how scrumptuous, succulent, sweet and sublime, can tranquilize us only temporarily. However, it is possible to discover the real cause of our appetite and then put together our own foodless recipe for lasting gratification.

When Do We Lose It? (Control, That Is)

We lose weight when we gain control effortlessly as the spontaneous result of insight—which, unfortunately, seems to be preceded by a lot of trial-and-error effort.

We gain weight most often when we're bored, stressed, fatigued, scared, hurt or angry, and when we don't have a clue to changing the way things are.

Where Do We Lose Control?

Rarely do we want to munch while we are building, making, creating. Compulsive eating happens most often during passive activities, often under the hypnotic influence of TV. Compulsive eaters are known by advertisers to be easily motivated to eat by outside stimuli.

Social activities and routine tasks both can trigger associations with food. Movies and sports, too. At church and family get-togethers, here comes more (of the most fattening) food.

With some people, just the sight of night—the end of the work day—sets off a series of impulses connected with extra eating, like a snack before bedtime or getting up in the middle of the night for a rendezvous in the kitchen with favorite calories.

Eating On The Road

For a compulsive eater, the most comfortable way to overeat is to eat out of sight, away from possible criticism from friends, family or even strangers. Secret eating takes many forms.

Corey: "Okay, I'm at least 50 pounds overweight and I know where it comes from, but I don't need to hear strangers commenting or laughing about how much I eat. So when I want lunch out, I pick places with drive-in windows. The person at the window doesn't know whether I'm ordering just for myself or for several people. Then

I eat in the car and don't have to wonder if some nosy person is counting my bags of French fries!"

Maureen: "I got into this habit of stopping at a convenience store on the way home from work. They have the same hard-to-find brand of cheese Danish I fell in love with while I was in the hospital, believe it or not. It's just great . . . of course, totally fattening—so soft and warm and melting when you put it in a microwave, and this store has a microwave. I do, too, of course, but this has become my own little private treat and I don't want it discussed at home. When I was in the hospital, I would dream about having this kind of cheese Danish the next morning for breakfast!

"Sometimes I drink milk with it—sometimes chocolate milk when I really feel like sinning all the way. It gives me something to look forward to all day long. Can't have it on weekends because the store is nearer my office and far from my home. It almost makes putting up with my job worth it! I don't even care that it's not quite what you'd usually have before dinner! Sometimes lately I've been having two."

Andy: "I've gotten so paranoid about people finding out how much I eat. I eat a lot in the car. I like to keep a tin of shortbread under the passenger seat. It just fits there and those things will keep a thousand years.

"But to show you how paranoid I've become, the other day I bought a carton of doughnuts on sale and was biting into one at a stop light when I sensed the driver beside me was staring at me. I actually took it out of my mouth and put it out of sight until he pulled away.

"The doughnuts, by the way, were a good buy but I had to eat them all before I got home so the deed wouldn't be discovered. Couldn't finish dinner as a result so I put some of it away until around 10:00. I can never sleep well when that happens."

Compulsive Hiding

Other ways to make others think we're eating less is to:

- Detour to the refrigerator on the way back from the bathroom at night.
- Stash food in our desks and chew quickly between reports.
- Generously volunteer to be the one to go for a take-out (then buy extra rolls to eat on the way home).
- "Forget" a meal-preparation essential at the market so we have an excuse to slip out for a tasty add-on treat.

All these ploys are the *modus operandi* of compulsive eaters. They use up time and energy but not calories—unless you are one of the many who designs a jogging route to include a yogurt store.

Much compulsive eating is hidden so that friends and families may suspect your weight situation is truly a physiological problem. They keep urging you to get it checked or would just rather assume it to be "genetic." (If you have any doubts, you certainly should meet with your doctor.)

You may find you hide things when you don't really need to—but you're embarrassed, so you hide anyway. Our shame can become so powerful that we even hide the reality of what we are doing from ourselves.

Many people for example, will prepare their own favorite dessert, faking themselves into thinking it is for family or friends. The sampling and tasting during cooking can easily become compulsive eating episodes. Like:

1. Making cookies for friends and eating so much of the dough that only enough is left for six (midget) cookies.
2. Baking a pie for the family and eating the whole thing before they even know of its existence. (This is based on the what-they-don't-know-won't-hurt-them school of foul food play.)
3. Dividing a dessert into "their part" and "my part" to hide any inequities created by an attack of compulsive eating.

Betraying our own generous instincts hurts and is just one of the many *icky* feelings that make compulsive eating not only a body problem but also an interference in our emotional lives. When our lack of control collides with what we want or should do for others, we are in deep water with our self-esteem. Only a thorough awareness of how we tripped into this muddle will lift the burden of guilt.

Profile Of A Compulsive Eater

If you are extremely frustrated over your lack of will-power when face-to-face with food, you are a compulsive eater. Self-discipline seems to be simple enough for other people when they are serious about making a change. They have what it takes to hold on to goals. For you, attempts at will power dissolve into a void where no goal really matters.

If you are a compulsive eater, a big chunk of every day is spent thinking about food—about eating it, about not eating it, about how much it's costing you physically, emotionally and financially, or just thinking about the weight you want to lose.

For many compulsive eaters, food is always in the fore-front of their minds. Before breakfast they're thinking about breakfast. After breakfast they're planning lunch and at lunch they may be talking about dinner—today's, yesterday's or tomorrow's.

This disturbing preoccupation with food can spill over into relationships. There is such pressure to deny we are out of control that we may go overboard in wanting to verify every tiny triumph in conversations about food with our friends. It's a tough friendship that can survive monologues like this: ". . . and then I had only one roll and I didn't put any butter on it, and then I had a salad with *miso* dressing, whatever that is, but I really wanted ranch, but I didn't give in, and then I had broiled chicken, not fried, and I turned down the mashed potatoes because who can eat them without lots of butter, and instead I had string beans, not my favorite but I had two helpings so I wouldn't be too interested in dessert, so then for dessert I had the very least worst, some sort of very light mousse, and I even left some—not a lot, but some. Then in my coffee I put . . ."

This preoccupation has another bad byproduct; it takes the edge off the love and happiness available to you now.

After tussling too long with conflicting desires, your physical energy has been worn down by frustration, fear, guilt and anger at yourself. How many years have you tried and failed? Reinforcing your sense of being a failure are your numerous vows of renewal. How many mornings have you awakened determined to quit, then by the afternoon all the old urges have taken over. Once again you are eating compulsively and saying to yourself, "I'm really going to get myself under control tomorrow."

Do you get angry with yourself over food? That's one of the worst features of compulsive eating. Each extra-eating episode carries the bad aftertaste of "I've failed again. I've let myself down again!" You endlessly reaffirm the negative messages about your capabilities: "What's wrong with me that I can't control myself?"

Weak, guilty, worthless—words that won't just go away. They are fed after every lost battle with The Urge, and although there are many other expressions of yourself that negate them, they return to haunt you every time you see your reflection. Body image remains a basic form of identification for every human being.

Good, Bad, Good, Bad

Our thoughts are either on the food we're going to eat or the food we're promising ourselves not to eat. A constant struggle. One day we think, "I've been good!" and then the next day it's, "I'm bad." Maybe the day begins with "good" and ends with "bad." Our entire sense of

Directions For The Functions Of Compulsive Eating Exercise:

Put yourself in the center. Put functions that compulsive eating have been serving in your life in the circle at the end of each arm. Write a sentence that describes the function identified in each arm. For example:

Function: Friendship (end of arm).
The sentence explaining it might read, "Food is the only friend I have."

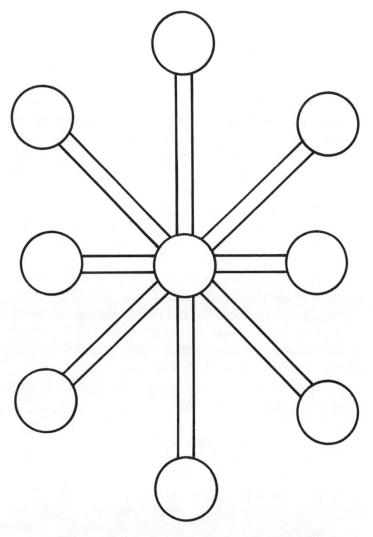

Figure 1. The Functions Of Compulsive Eating

self-worth becomes based on how we've handled The Urge from day to day, hour to hour.

Constantly we're trying to gain control and not eat. Yet the Other Side takes over. Soon, we know we've lost our resolve and we're eating again. Then come the thoughts and feelings of disappointment and depression.

However, we are hardly alone in this. Similarly, we were not alone at the time we began incorporating into our deepest selves the need for this way out of an otherwise intolerable emotional impasse. (To better understand what overeating now means to you, see Figure 1.) When we are thoroughly "fed up" with the dysfunctional solution represented by compulsive eating, we won't be alone, either, as we leave it behind. We will join with many others who are finding the awareness it takes, who are practicing new behaviors and trying on new ways of looking at themselves, their past and their future.

Monica

I cannot handle any more diets. They are so painful. I went from BaylorFast to Weight Watchers to Pritikin, then to grapefruit, then Nutri-System, then Doctor's Quick Weight Loss and back to fasting, then back to Weight Watchers, then weight-loss pills, high protein diet and high carbohydrate diet. I've been dieting for 15 years and am so frustrated.

A lot of my problem comes from my fear of being alone. When my husband goes out of town, I eat Twinkies. Twinkies keep me company. I couldn't eat them when I was younger because my mother wouldn't buy them for me. She said they were totally void of nutrition, which of course they are, but it wasn't as though I wanted to eat Twinkies and nothing else, for God's sake. She wouldn't let me have one, ever.

So now I feel I'm really giving something to myself. I can get away with eating them. No one knows. They help me think about something other than how lonely I feel. Twinkies sedate me, only I don't feel good physically afterwards because of all that sugar.

An Affirmation To Stop Compulsive Eating
And Start Healthy Living

At the end of each chapter you'll find reality reminders like the following to reinforce what the Inner You knows to be true. You might want to copy them into a notebook that can be your companion during the times of doubt we all face.

I choose to make my life what I want it to be. I take the time to learn about myself and my needs in order to create vibrant health. I have the courage to change whatever I need to change in my life. Every day I am learning new ways to make myself safe without using food or fat.

TWO

Permanent Weight Reduction: Are You Really Ready?

Compulsive eating develops as a means of coping with life when we can't see a better way out.

We learn our coping skills in childhood. If, in these especially formative years, we aren't helped over the rough spots with better means for surviving difficult times—or if we have somehow been deprived of the psychological fortitude to handle tough situations—we may take comfort in food.

After we've put some years behind us and our eating "solution" has resulted in new chronic problems associated with weight, we begin to realize that eating only numbs the pain very temporarily and that, meanwhile, no magic solutions have appeared to take away the hurts behind the munching.

Waiting For The Wizard Of Oz

Magic—that's what we all hope for at various times in our lives when we simply are stumped over our situations.

Maybe we will meet someone accidentally while shopping for motor oil, or a registerd letter will arrive from sweepstakes headquarters, or the office ogre will be bitten by a rabid squirrel. Magic has happened to all of us at one time or another; maybe if we just sit tight (with perhaps a bag of mesquite-flavored jalapeno ruffled potato chips) it will strike at the core of our miseries.

And, then, maybe not.

If you're really ready for permanent weight loss and have had it with seesawing up and down on diets of various sorts, you won't fight the idea that you may have to start making your own magic in the area of your life where compulsive eating has taken over.

Fed Up Enough?

Consider: Have you really had it—or are you just experiencing another round of remorse? Any chronic problem takes a giant size helping of motivation for an individual to stay with the often uncomfortable processes of change. That's Change with a capital C. We're not talking here about switching from sugar to sorbitol or climbing onto some shiny chrome machine that costs as much as Jane Fonda's public appearances. For compulsive eaters, turning away from the table when extra eating is involved requires turning their lives around. And that takes a commitment not just to looking and feeling better but to doing some things that, at first, are going to feel a lot less comfortable than opening a refrigerator door. They are going to be activities we may have managed to avoid.

Weight Loss Equals Happiness vs. Happiness Equals Weight Loss

For the first five years of her job as circulation manager of a daily business paper, Jenine was in love with her work. The long hours were equal to the satisfaction she found in developing herself professionally. But then the job became fairly routine, problems arose with management and a good friend at work left. There was nothing dramatically wrong but the edge had gone from her enthusiasm. She whittled the hours down to a more normal schedule, yet when she got home to her husband, a comedy writer, there wasn't much *joie de vivre* to share with him. She was terminally bored. Her listlessness put her to sleep in front of the television night after night — for five more years.

"Absolutely the most excitement I had during the last two years was a fried banana pastry or a custard-layered cake every afternoon. I ordered them take-out from a Thai restaurant and they were exquisite. And a box of *petit fours* I bought once a week. It went from eight ounces to a pound and a half a week in two years. I went from a size 12 to an 18 in the same period."

Jenine's husband repeatedly urged her, in heated arguments that didn't help their marriage, to make a serious move toward employment elsewhere. Her initiatives, though, seldom went further than responding, several days after they appeared, to a few ads for what she had already decided she didn't want to do anymore.

"I just hate job-hunting—fixing up the resume differently for different positions, the interviews, waiting. And I really don't know what I want. Staying put seems less stressful for now."

No matter how much weight she lost temporarily during various diets she tried at this time, a slimmer figure didn't make her job less boring. Until she made the commitment to either intensify her job hunting efforts or to find out what was behind her reluctance to improve her life, boredom would remain to prompt extra eating. With the help of a therapist she was able to examine where the misunderstood grounds for her lack of self-worth came from. Her new perceptions gave her the energy and confidence to change her unsatisfactory life—and her extra appetite for snacking vanished.

Another Way We're Like Gorillas

Compulsive eating can be an escape from the question of what to do with your time to make your life more stimulating. Compulsive eating can become your main stimulation. Researchers of animal behavior have shown that gorillas languishing in zoos where adequate stimulation is missing will also overeat and get fat, sit around, mope and become depressed. One female gorilla in particular gained so much weight she could barely climb up the structures built for her.

Humans have a tremendous need for stimulation in their lives, too. They can tolerate sameness just so long, then need to be refreshed with new professional challenges, a new hobby, a change of scene, new friends, other recreation.

Eating often is used to quell the boredom of routine relationships and avoid the risk of trying something new. It's easy to get locked into humdrum situations, with spouses especially, that can become boring. If spouses are working, we wish they were home. Yet once they are, we do the same things over and over until they become mechanical. (We know we must be having fun because the first time we did it, six years ago, it was fun!) There's a lot going on inside everyone but relationships can seem routine when new ways to bring out different thoughts and feelings aren't tried.

Trying new things out—often they don't feel easy or natural when you've become a creature of erroneous eating habits. But if you are fed up enough with waiting for magical solutions—if the reality of unwanted weight and its attendant problems is weighing too much on your mind—you may have what it takes for permanent weight loss: serious motivation.

Ambivalence: Is Thin Really Me Any More?

Repeatedly while working with people who are struggling to lose weight, I have noticed within them a certain ambivalence. When attempting to break the compulsive eating cycle and lose weight, most people experience internal conflict. They definitely want to lose weight, yet . . . just beneath the surface there is ambivalence which is often unexpressed. This is especially evident when they remain at a certain weight for a long time in spite of all their efforts at dieting.

You can make your own assessment of the purpose of fat in your life with The Functions Of My Fat exercise (see Fig. 2). Draw your face or your figure in the center. In each of as many circles as you need, put a function that fat has been serving in your life. In the pathway leading from you to your function circle, write a sentence describing the function.

For example, if you write "True Friendship" in a circle, the pathway might read, "I attract friends who look beyond appearances."

A woman attorney I know felt that extra pounds became a professional asset. She was quite frank about her shape and had made peace with the likelihood that her attitude toward her body would never result in substantial weight loss.

"I use my weight, " she confessed, "to be big and intimidating. It bolsters me up and helps me look mean and formidable.

"In law school I got psyched out by the tough guys in my class and doubted whether anyone would take a *little girl* like me seriously. That's what my father called me at age 22—his 'little girl.' But I wanted to be a litigator and little girls aren't hired as litigators.

"I had started to gain weight in law school after I got married and was away from my family and friends for the first time. I didn't have time to make good meals, exercise or anything except study. Which, of course, was very stressful. I grabbed at junk food and gained.

"I was amazed at how different I started looking as I became a 'fat person' but I didn't consider it a permanent condition until I realized it was making me behave differently. I really felt more substantial, like more of a pres-

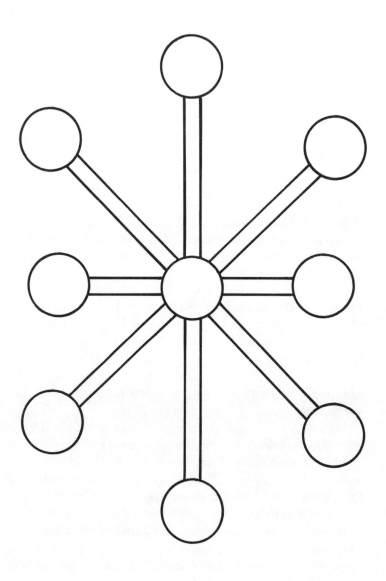

Figure 2. The Function Of My Fat

ence in that mock courtroom we used at law school. Whether or not it was because of my appearance, I felt people treated me with more respect, not like the frivolous female I always dreaded being perceived as. And since I was short, to boot, I needed this, although I still continued to give lip service to losing. I still really believed I wanted to lose."

This woman's subconscious mind had an agenda other than weight loss. The fear of being thin or attractive was working against her achieving a weight that was healthy. The benefits of losing weight did not outweigh those of keeping it on. Being the protective mechanism that it is, the subconscious cooperated by helping her avoid change and thereby escape what she perceived to be the lukewarm advantages of thinness.

Ultimately, she came to recognize that, unconsciously, she had been using her weight, her size, to bolster her confidence and establish boundaries she knew no other way to achieve. She paid a high price for this means of self-enhancement and protection, but it worked, and she was not about to give it up. Her efforts at weight reduction were sabotaged.

The Meaning Of Weight

Self-confidence and boundaries are necessary to get ahead and to avoid being walked over. Building self-regard and acquiring effective skills for communicating feelings take time but do not create the health and social limitations of excessive weight.

Dorin, a collections representative for an air cargo carrier before she went back home to live, was surprised at the length of the list she gave me in response to the following sentence I asked her to complete:

As long as I stay fat I don't have to:

• Be in the dating scene.
• Worry about being rejected.

- Look perfect all the time.
- Wonder why I don't get promoted.
- Get up and do things I don't want to do.
- Take care of myself.
- Work really hard at staying slim.
- Set limits for myself.
- Protect myself.
- Tell people to leave me alone.
- Expose my body.
- Spend time with people I don't want to be with.
- Put myself "out there."
- Get married.
- Be perfect.
- Do anything.

This exercise clearly revealed to her the ambivalence she felt regarding losing weight.

Ambivalence creates an inner conflict that is paralyzing and prevents any positive action.

Another way to explore your feelings in this area is to notice obese and thin people and pay attention to your reactions. What do you think to yourself when you see a thin woman walking next to a fat one? Chances are you feel more openness toward the overweight person.

To find out what you've been telling yourself about fat and thin, try the same exercise I give participants in my compulsive eating groups. On a sheet of paper, make two lists of completed sentences beginning with "Thin is . . ." and "Fat is . . ." Then compare your responses with the following set given by Carey, a gorgeous redhead disguised by 200 pounds of weight she thought was a complete negative until she made this inventory.

Carey's Fat And Thin List

Thin Is . . .

Positive	Negative	Positive & Negative
Beautiful	Threatening	Sexual
Getting all the breaks	Not flexible	Taking and not giving
Good	Controlling	Powerful
In control	Self-centered	Well-disciplined
Self-caring	Cold	Having it all
People gravitate to her	Bitch	Selfish
Popular	Not using brains	Having all the men
Fun	Not working very hard	
Charismatic	Not fun	
	Aloof	
	Being paranoid about staying thin	
	Manipulative	

Fat Is . . .

Positive	Negative	Positive & Negative
Fun	Repulsive	Vulnerable
Casual	Sick	
Giving	Dumpy, frumpy	
Nurturing	Dumb, not bright	
Mothering	Asexual	
Approachable	Lonely	
Non-threatening	Hungry	
Sensitive	No self-control	
Caring	Doesn't think about self	
Considerate		
Compassionate		

It is vital to release the associations we have with fat and thin in order to break the compulsive eating cycle.

We come to recognize that it isn't the fat or lack of fat on one's body which determines internal nature.

A thin person can be fun, nurturing, approachable, sensitive and caring. A fat person can be querulous, cold, self-centered and not fun.

We let our hearts determine our nature, not our fat.

Making Changes Requires Making Time

To quit compulsive eating and harboring fat, you must have the commitment to set aside time for yourself. Perhaps you have bitten off more projects than you can chew or you have reluctantly committed what might be extra time to doing for others. You might have to ask that these hours be returned to you. If you tend to be the sort of soft-hearted victim who can't say *no* and certainly can't stand the thought of someone scowling at you, you may find ideas for reclaiming time for reading, talking out your feelings, meditating and exercising in a later chapter.

Our priorities have to be reordered if we're on a tight schedule. Eating is a quick fix; redirecting our lives takes time. We must come to a strong sense that all lives are worth setting straight—especially our own!

We can learn how to expand our sense of self-worth so that we project the attitude we want. We don't have to use a padded body to do it for us. The attitudes we broadcast act as an energy field that others perceive, although it is not visible. When our boundaries are established by our healthy mental and physical energies, we gain respect and recognition from those around us.

As long as we are lugging around superfluous fat, we can't become aware of the genuine power that we have within. We are withholding knowledge of an important and impressive part of ourselves.

Tricia

I resent society's saying we're supposed to look this way or that. I guess a part of me is staying fat to rebel against how others expect me to be. I don't have to live in a perfect body. I'm too much of a perfectionist in the rest of my life, anyway. Eating is sort of a release from all this for me.

I've always felt, anyway, like I'm on the outside looking in. I mean, I've always been fat and I want to look slim, although the thought of being on the inside or looking slim is kind of scary. Often I see thin women and think they look conceited or absorbed in their looks and I feel I don't want to look that way because other people will then think I'm like that, too.

Still, I would like my children to have a skinnier mom.

An Affirmation To Stop Compulsive Eating And To Start Healthy Living

I no longer need food or fat to help me cope with life. I release any need I may have to limit my health and happiness through eating and carrying excess fat. I am learning to set limits in my world and take time for myself. Effortlessly, I convince others of who I am without weight.

THREE

Where To Begin To End Dieting

Love food?

Silly question.

So when we deprive ourselves of something we love every time we go on a diet, it's no wonder weight-loss programs fail to hold our interest.

To stop eating compulsively, you must first stop depriving yourself.

Say what?

Yes, dieting guarantees PDD—Post Diet Depression — and subsequent weight gain for most compulsive eaters. Every overweighter is well qualified to direct and star in a professional quality horror movie titled, of course, "Return of the Flab." Where it goes, no one knows. Where it comes from we all know too well. It doesn't matter whether we've lost a little or a lot, it catches up with most of us sooner or later.

A jazz singer and piano player popular in Miami nightclubs was featured in a newspaper's Sunday magazine article for his astounding change in appearance after he went on a well-known diet program. It was a tribute to his nationally recognized talents that he became, prior to the diet, successful in such a competitive field despite his profound burden of fat. His weight exceeded 300 pounds, distinctive facial features obliterated by the commonality of obese roundness. Nor did he dress in any distinctive way to glamorize the mother lode of calories he consumed daily.

After the diet—which was supplemented by surgery — he looked like American Gigolo. A lean, well-proportioned body and a film star's—no, a model's—handsomeness had been hidden under the mounds of fat.

And soon to be hidden again.

In less than a year, readers of the paper in which his triumph over the tyranny of compulsive eating had been detailed were horrified to learn that his inspiring story had gone into reverse. After all that effort—all the talk, all the gustatory denial, all the expense, surgery, new wardrobe, new publicity photos, pride of accomplishment, attention, praise—virtually all of the fat was back.

"The look just wasn't me," he said. "Being thin didn't feel that comfortable."

Other public figures of greater and lesser reputations have gone the same route. It wasn't enough that thousands, millions, of people would become aware of their failure. In some instances, their careers were on the line. A need deeper and more essential than the approval of society—or of themselves—derailed their efforts.

No More Dieting

The novelty wears off. Your stamina and enthusiasm wane. On the inside, you feel as though you're starving. Your habit has been to reward yourself with food when you do well. Now there are no rewards. There's a void where before there was an excited, gratified feeling.

Who needs THIS?

Aware Indulgence

A stepping stone to permanent weight loss used by many people with success is Aware Indulgence.

One of the best ways to start losing weight permanently: Eat whatever, whenever.

This isn't the road-to-nowhere contradiction it appears to be. First, to work, it must follow two acknowledgments made with conviction:

- We have a problem that dieting can never resolve.
- Deprivation isn't the answer; it's part of the problem.

"I acknowledge, I acknowledge," you say, "now pass the chocolate chip cookies—and what's the catch?"

Okay. If there were absolutely no internal or external restrictions on how many you could eat in a day—no guilt whatsoever—how many could you handle? Five, a dozen, two dozen? Place your order—the catch is that every step of the eating process has to be done with as much awareness as you can muster to really feel what you are doing and what effect food truly has on you, mentally and physically.

Much overeating is a mechanical process with just the initial mouthfuls being truly enjoyable and the remainder of the experience a desperate, joyless and numbing activity, totally psychological in nature, hitching a ride on those first fun bites.

This exercise begins to restore our ability to be sensitive to every aspect of compulsive eating and its origins. It will take patience with ourselves to observe rather than mechanically mask what we have been doing because not wanting to look at something painful is at the very foundation of compulsive eating.

This first step in our new way of observing will begin convincing us that there are valid alternative ways to look at what we and others do and have done. With this simple beginning, we will start exploring the notion that our old ways of seeing weren't the only ways to see. We will find there are other ways of observing our world that weren't known either by our young selves or by our early mentors, who were themselves unavoidably in the dark about different ways to react to what life is about.

The consequences of the new way we will be looking at old hurts will be very different from the downward spiral into compulsive eating that we once had no choice but to take.

The Month It Rained Cupcakes:
A Personal Experiment

At one time I was in an unrelenting battle with cupcakes: I need you, I don't need you, I want you, I can do without you, etc. Every day after work I stopped and bought a bunch to eat on the way home. Soon, I felt like I was a pawn of cupcakes. I hated myself, of course, for not being able to resist their puffy little charms.

Finally I had to make the inevitable comparison that virtually all of us make at one time or another: I felt like a drug addict who needed a fix every day, my self-esteem dipping lower and lower. Maybe it was cute that my fix was "just" cupcakes but the added weight didn't look cute.

Then, at some point, after trying unsuccessfully, as always, to psyche myself out of the cupcake habit, I decided to experiment with giving in. So I had to have those cupcakes, did I? Well, then, I'd stop splitting myself in two by claiming, on one hand, that they were vital to enjoying my day, then on the other hand, scolding myself that they weren't. They couldn't be both, and my actions showed more than my words what I really believed about me and cupcakes.

All right, I was weak and dependent and I would buy as many as I wanted and stop pretending I was someone else. I would retreat from the battlefield, surrender, quit feeling guilty and enjoy. I gave myself permission to have them without chastising myself. I was only human.

Every day I eagerly went to the store, loaded up with cupcakes and then made a ritual of eating them. Essential to this was slowing down and tasting every bite.

The first time, I was in Cupcake Heaven. It was an unforgettably self-indulgent experience, the likes of which I must not have had since age ten. I wasn't eating any more than the excess I had become accustomed to, but odd things began to happen.

The taste changed. The first time I noticed this I thought I'd just bought a bad package. But through the following days a plastic-like taste grew stronger. They also began feeling too heavy, too rich. They landed with a thud in my stomach. Next reaction, and the most alarming, was the sensation of sugar spreading through my system. What was happening to me?

The answer: nothing more than usual, except now I was focusing on the entire experience. I was not just mechanically munching my way through to the end, hypnotized by the initial rush of gratification, minimizing or blocking the negatives. All of these reactions had happened to me many times before but then I was not totally tuned in. Now that I was, I could see that refusing to look at all the effects of binges on my body and mind was a symptom of a deeper "seeing" disability in my life.

We need to acquire the strength to lift up the rugs of our life and see what emotions have been swept underneath. We acquire this strength by discovering and practicing healthier ways of observing ourselves and others.

Overdo It!

I didn't give up cupcakes so easily, though. I found it hard to believe that these little goodies that had added spice to my days were no longer lifting me up. Instead, they started bringing me down. I gave them several more chances, as long as The Urge persisted.

One historic day, when The Urge hit hard, I was recalling how my body felt after eating them. It was not just the quickly dismissed remembrance that I sometimes had before, but a very vivid memory of the fully experienced reactions of Cupcake Month.

I passed the store.

Once in a while after that, I went back, but the spell was broken. The habit was gone. There was no more guilt or self-hate fueling my urge. I was free to examine what was really happening.

One day, a few months later, I realized that I hadn't thought about cupcakes in a long time.

I discovered that a part of me — a small part, at that — had sold the rest of me a bill of goods on cupcake binging. All along, the biggest part of me was surviving my unfulfilled needs, despite cupcakes, by myself. Cupcake comfort was just an exercise in self-hypnosis, like a placebo with undesirable side effects, creating more problems than it solved.

Reading this exercise and doing it yourself is the difference between looking at a postcard and being there. Take a multi-dimensional trip into your most forbidden food (**with your physician's consent** if problems with sugar and carbohydrate binging may exist). It can be a significant start at freeing yourself from the tyranny of forbidden food.

Weight gain is common in this phase as you experience the relief and exhilaration of not dieting. This is usually accompanied by panic and fear that you are out of control, that guilt-free compulsive eating could go on forever. It's vital to hang in there, not go near the scales and not seek refuge in another diet out of terror that this experiment will never end.

Your Need Begins To Change

Giving in with guilt perpetuates compulsive eating. Giving in without guilt is the beginning of a befriending process in which you replace condemnation, self-hate and a dysfunctional method of coping with understanding and appreciation. As you develop your dormant powers of awareness, you'll one day find the urge to respond to your body's need for health more compelling than the urge to feed your emotional needs with food.

It will just happen — not while you are anxiously waiting for change but because you have given up thinking and worrying about it. You are involved in doing something positive about compulsive eating.

Naturally — without a sense of deprivation — you'll find yourself folding up the bag or box of junk food with plenty left inside. Without forcing or deprivation, you just won't want the portions you previously craved. You'll feel full longer, find yourself skipping ritual snack times. You'll acquire the ability to eat small quantities of sweets without going overboard. And you will develop cravings for foods other than sweets.

The Next Plateau

However, don't think you're going to get off that easily. Your weight will begin stabilizing as the binging fades by itself. Then it will start to drop. Just as you feel you have finally taken the bull by the horns, depression sets in.

The emotions previously suppressed by all that food you've grown tired of begin to surface. This is the stage where therapy, journaling (experiencing your thoughts in concrete form via an informal diary) or talking with friends become critical. Don't be misled into thinking that you can sidestep one or all of these helps. If you are reluctant, experiment with setting aside that reluctance. Nothing is more valuable than an experimental spirit when the need for change is obvious. You have nothing to lose

lose but your weight since you are not obliged to continue with anything that doesn't feel comfortable. That's what dumping deprivation was all about.

The Compulsive Eater's Bill of Rights

We Hold These Truths To Be Self-Validating:

We have the right to not lose or to lose.
We have the right to gain or to not gain.
We have the right to change not at all, a little or substantially.
We have the right to try, back off, try something else.
We have the right to think like we've never thought before because we see as we've never seen before.
We have the right to learn who we were before and who we are today.

Sense The Power

As you gain control over food and it no longer controls you, a sense of power arises. You acquire the ability to replace eating for other noninjurious pleasures. Some of these might include getting involved in new activities, establishing new friendships, reading, taking naps or going for walks. You begin to eliminate seeing yourself in ways that are related to food or your body. You talk less about food and weight. You are more patient with your relapses because you have the knowledge that you are neither more nor less human than anyone else.

The new ability to distinguish physical hunger from emotional hunger has grown. This growth has made it less possible to fool ourselves that filling up the stomach fills up the heart.

Donna's Cupcake Diary

Day 1: I feel like school let out for the summer, like I was just released from food prison. All the cupcakes I can eat? Whee!

Day 2: I'm going to get so fat but I trust the process. Such freedom from anxiety. I feel lighter inside.

Day 3: Won't have quite so many today. I am tempted to feel guilt but can't because it's just an experiment. I have the power to end it at any time. Let's see what happens.

Day 4: Now that the child in me has been allowed to run free, I'm getting messages that maybe, on its own, it wants to change what it's doing. Don't want to eat as many as on Day 1.

Day 5: I've discovered a vaguely artificial quality to these cupcakes. A sort of preservative taste in the background I'd never noticed. Wonder if rats or something in laboratories have died from this stuff.

Day 6: Shelf life of these things has got to be at least 100 years. They're starting to feel too rich. I left half of one uneaten.

Day 7: These cupcakes must be aging me rapidly. I never used to have this sensation afterwards. Feels like I've got a baggie of playdough lodged in my digestive track.

Day 8: I'm noticing a sugar rush and an uncomfortable buzzing in my head. It's as though I can actually feel the sugar entering my bloodstream. There's no history of negative reaction to sugar in my family . . . what's happening to me?

An Affirmation To Stop Compulsive Eating And Start Healthy Living

I accept myself as I am today. I am compassionate and gentle with myself as I grow and change. I accept all of myself. I do things to make myself happy. Every day I take the time to tune in to my needs and take care of myself. I now have the desire to tune in to my body and befriend it. I listen to it and it tells me the truth. The truth sets me free to feel better and live better.

FOUR

Identifying Your
Body Blocks

The human body, it's true, is a marvelous machine. In fact, we might complain, it can be too marvelous.

It keeps a perfect record of our personal history and beliefs, including everything we may try to forget on a conscious level.

It stores the records of all our past traumas and neglect. These stored experiences, rather than being buried deep in ooze-proof vaults within our subconscious, go into leaky containers. They overflow from our brains into our bodies and there show up as fat, muscle tension or negative postures.

Emotionally, these blocks are often experienced as fatigue, depression, lethargy or sluggishness. They depress the entire physical and emotional system. Lack of drive and motivation is the result. These blocks can greatly impact on compulsive eating.

Lethargy and fatigue provide high-octane fuel for eating episodes.

That is why the end of the working day is such a difficult time for compulsive eaters. Moreover, if you have
body blocks, you may already be running at half your
capacity. You are then more likely to be tired and eat
compulsively after work or other stressful periods.

Mirror Therapy

Since body blocks can be one of the underlying reasons
for fat accumulation, recognizing these blocks and releasing them is an important part of the total healing picture.
The best place to begin this process is in the privacy of
your own home right in front of the (gulp!) mirror.

Look at your body in a full-length mirror. For some of
us this may take heroic courage. But that's a good way to
become your own hero. You'll be amazed how much you'll
look up to yourself when you've permanently outgrown
compulsive eating. A hint: It's easier if you examine your
reflection with objective, even clinical, realism rather than
with your emotional side; there are many others who will
see a very similar shape, arrived at in very similar ways.
Letting go of your personal identification with a fat body
is part of losing your fat. You can be fat, but you can be
other than fat, too — if you think the time has come. Fat
isn't the only shape you can make yourself and still be you.

Try to withhold judgment as you study your mirror
image. You didn't invent compulsive eating. It's a wide-
spread, very human and often "taught" means of coping.

Look at the parts of your body that have accumulated
pounds on them or are out of shape.

Notice your posture and where you feel the greatest
tension. You can learn a great deal about your unmet needs
by tuning in to what you see. There are several body
blocks represented by the shapes of compulsive eaters.

The Compassion Bend

The physical characteristics of the Compassion Bend
include slumping shoulders which roll forward. This pos-

ture gives a slightly caved-in look to the chest and creates
the impression that the person is trying to protect a soft,
vulnerable part. This could point up depression from an
unhappy childhood. Or it could be the result of carrying
other people's burdens. Sometimes it is the physical manifestation of an unconscious attempt to hide sexuality.

A particular type of family background may be an underlying factor with body blocks such as the Compassion
Bend. It symbolizes a desire to wrap around, protect, join
with and help others. Research by Dr. Harriet Bachner-
Schnorr has shown that adult children of alcoholics, for
example, tend to be more intuitive and sensitive than the
general population. This is also true of many compulsive
eaters. Many of us came from alcoholic or dysfunctional
families. We feel things deeply. If you have this type of
personal history you may be viewed by others as a nice,
caring person who is easy to get along with. You may
have a tendency to be other-centered. You probably give
more than you receive.

Therapists, physicians and healers of all kinds often
take on the Compassion Bend posture unconsciously.

Fortunately, it is possible to be sensitive, intuitive and
an excellent helper without having the Compassion Bend.
To "unbend," we may need to resolve some issues from
our past and learn to care for others without usurping
responsibilities rightly their own.

People with the Compassion Bend usually have a powerful nurturing ability which is used freely with others
and sparingly with themselves. The nurturing parent within all of us must be allowed to flower fully and that means
being given adequate time to attend to its closest "next of
kin," or Inner Child — the one who wants the cookie
when its needs aren't met.

Weight Of The World

This body block begins with the rolled or slumped
shoulders and is further emphasized by sagging facial fea-

tures, a burdensome walk or morbid obesity. If this applies
to you, you probably are worried about the needs of others
and have a lot of fear inside. Perhaps your concern for
others is shown by suffering yourself. You use food to
ease this pain.

The Crustaceans

Their appearance hasn't changed for a zillion years.
Their houses look the same and their clothes are usually
old and worn, sometimes with holes that "don't matter."
They have not updated themselves for a very long time
and may have a hair style dating back a few decades.

Their body type is obese and out of shape. Eating is one
of the only pleasures they get from life and their bodies
show it. They sometimes have a waddle or slow, laboring
gait. Their posture and movement give the impression
that they are indeed carrying a shell on their back, many
years in the making, which is hard to lug around.

Revitalization of the entire system is needed to resolve
the Crustacean problem. Learning how the world can be
trusted and reaching out to explore it is essential. Caught
at the red light of past traumas, they can't move on until
the light changes. Trouble is, they control the green light
switch. Only they have the power to resolve old misper-
ceptions and start practicing healthy self-nurturance.

Their shell exists only to protect their soft, vulnerable
inner selves. The strength that comes from health, self-
awareness and effective boundary setting provides much
better protection which is lighter and easier to carry. Compulsive eating subsides as their life broadens and they
develop other interests.

Catcher's Shield

This is a male block, generally. Its common physical characteristics are a distended stomach that balloons over
pants. People with Catcher's Shields usually work hard and

keep long hours. They take care of everybody else's needs but don't seem to know how to have fun. Their primary pleasures in life are eating and, for some, drinking.

This body block is potentially very dangerous. Fat collecting on the stomach area will put pressure on the heart and could contribute to a heart attack. A man with this condition probably grew up in a rough world which was insensitive to his needs and feelings. As a result, he wears his shield-like catcher's belly to protect him from the insensitivity around him.

This man often appears gruff, shows no feelings and is domineering. He probably works in a cold, unfeeling environment where he has to act tough even when he doesn't feel tough on the inside. He may live in an isolated world. He is as hidden and protected as a baseball catcher in full gear. Nobody gets in — except food — and he doesn't come out and show himself. Since the solar plexus is the area where feelings are received, this is the area which is the most sensitive to the outside world. The catcher's belly shield protects him from blows and keeps him safe inside.

Integration of the inside person and the outside person is needed for resolution of this problem. New information about the self and others is required to restore a more relaxed and natural personality, attracting "safe" relationships and allowing the body's safety gear to be dropped. This is a dynamic, exciting process that also releases any excessive sense of responsibility for the lives of others. What at first seemed unessential — more time for play, more time for fun and more disclosure of personal emotions to others — becomes sensible and necessary for change.

Compulsive eating subsides as we learn healthier ways to protect ourselves, reducing the need for fat as armor.

Hey, Babe

Whatever happened to Baby Jane (or John)?

Back to the mirror. What do you see now that you wouldn't have seen when you were, say, five months old?

Among other things, the purity of your baby spirit was there for all to see as reflected in every part of an infant's body. Somewhere inside you is recorded the memory of the time when you naturally felt good in your skin — relaxed, joyous and fun, stretching and feeling yourself with the pleasure of simply existing. Yet somehow in the process of growing up, the best of our babyhood was covered over with the techniques of survival in a confusing world.

You weren't born hating your body, comparing it to others or eating compulsively. The disassociation from, or disowning of, your body happened through years of stored traumas. Often we lose our innocence and learn to feel bad about our bodies because of the burdens we unconsciously picked up from others. Many people, too, who were abused as children displaced to their own bodies the hate they felt toward the molester they depended on. So let's experiment when we look into that mirror. Go back to scratch, back to basics:

- Without that body you see in the mirror — regardless of its condition — existence on this plane is impossible.
- Our bodies are the only real homes we have, our only reliable transportation.
- We should forgive our bodies as much as they forgive us. Our bodies are amazingly forgiving. They are our best supporters, always striving to right the wrongs we perpetrate on them.

These are all excellent reasons to ease up when we look in that mirror. Allowing ourselves those old feelings of disgust and hopelessness when we catch sight of the fat on our bodies often makes us feel that the road to remodeling is too long. So, out of desperation, we succumb to another eating episode.

Coming to accept and love the body you have right now is essential to the healing process.

The Blocked Inner Child

All body blocks result from past deprivation. Within each one of us blocked compulsive eaters is an adaptive, frightened child who never was satisfied emotionally, a child who is in desperate need of a loving, nurturing parent. This parent waits inside only to be recognized. Inside us all is an Inner Parent, that aspect of ourselves that is able to draw limits and establish protective boundaries for us.

This nurturing parent can be compassionate and loving to the world but at the same time protective of the vulnerable Inner Child. As a result, the child inside is no longer overburdened, beaten down with discouragement or living in emotional poverty. It has permission to breathe freely and be happy. The internal parent took the responsibility for making a safe world in which the Inner Child can live comfortably.

Body-blocked adults had thwarted childhoods. There was no one there providing adequate support for our innocence, playfulness and beauty. As children we had to be little adults, losing the intuitive knowledge of how to play and be light. Now, playing as an adult feels all wrong to us but our life experience still remains in the red in that place at our center where the psychological accounts are kept. There is a debt that demands to be paid but we've been programmed for guilt. We feel more secure having body blocks to shield us from adding to our "sins," taking what we think we don't deserve. This security soon becomes misery, however, because body blocks eventually stifle all growth and development.

There are a number of areas of exploration, plus exercises, that can be done to release these blocks and get the flow of energy moving again. Freely flowing energy in the body revitalizes and rejuvenates. Some of the areas we will be exploring later in this book that will trigger releases for you include the role of the family in eating disorders, reparenting yourself and springing the anger trap.

Befriending Your Body

So many people I've seen over the years have expressed a hatred for their bodies, describing them as "gross," "ugly" and "disgusting." Often, this has absolutely nothing to do with the actual size of their bodies. Some women who are five pounds overweight will talk about their legs as "huge" or their stomach as "poochy." One woman, a citrus grower, said her body was "as big as a barn."

This total rejection of body is dangerous to psychological and physical health. The subconscious is always listening to your thoughts and feelings about yourself. Many researchers have shown in studies that this negativity can determine the state of health in the body. In a longevity study, Dr. Paul Pearsal, author of *Superimmunity*, noted that his participants who reported themselves in good or excellent condition — not always an accurate self-assessment — did live longer than those who reported themselves as being in poor health whether or not they actually were.

When our lives are stressed beyond our ability to cope, we have a tendency to engage in self-destructive thoughts and behaviors, often resulting in what Pearsal has called "autocerebral disease." Some of these behaviors include compulsive eating, eating high-fat foods, smoking, drinking or even driving without a seat belt.

Disliking or hating your body is a prerequisite for abusing it. This self-abuse, frequently unnoticed, will continue unchecked.

Test yourself for self-abuse. It's the crime of the century!

Pick a day, any day, and keep pad and pen with you throughout. Every time you give yourself an abusive message, whether it's about your body, your mind, your "luck," or your potential, note it. Every time you abuse yourself with food, overwork, lack of rest or other neglect, that deserves a notation, too. Be frank, be alert and you'll be astounded at the negative self-programming to which you're subjected. This dawning awareness is healing, one of the many forms of awareness-expansion available to you that can change your perspective on your body, yourself and your life.

A Visualization For Positive Body Image

Here's an exercise to help you see your way to a slimmer body. It is recommended that you do it once a day for 30 days. It helps curb compulsive eating while strengthening a clear, positive image of yourself with a lean, fit body. In order for visualizations to work best, you must see the image you create clearly and recall it often.

Begin by sitting or lying in a comfortable position in a place where there are no distractions. It is important that you completely relax, let go and experience.

First, **take a few deep breaths,** allowing the air to enter and fill your lungs, lifting your collarbone. On the exhale, breathe out all the stress and tension of the day, letting the "busy-ness" slide away. Allow your body to go completely limp as you feel yourself relaxing. As you do so, remain completely alert. On each in-breath, you are rejuvenated with life, feeling light with heightened awareness. As you continue to breathe, bring yourself into focused attention for this visualization exercise.

Next, **see yourself standing in the middle of a room** which is flooded with sunlight. It has bright shining floors and a large full-length mirror on the wall. As you stand in the room, **picture yourself as separate from your excess weight.** Imagine this weight to be a cloak you've been wearing around you. See yourself taking off this cloak, slipping it from your shoulders and dropping it behind you on the floor. With it you have taken off everything that has been weighing you down.

Immediately you feel new life and energy. You stand in front of the full length mirror and **notice your slim, fit body.** You feel good, while enjoying how your body looks. Notice that your neck looks longer and your shoulders are easy to hold up as you stand up straight. You look down and your thighs are smooth and firm. Your legs appear longer. They are strong and lean and you feel as though you would have the spring of a gazelle.

You **continue scanning your body** and notice your stomach. It is flat and tight and your hip bones are showing, giving a beautiful curvature to the stomach area. You are aware that it feels good to be in your body. You feel proud, accepting and thankful for the beautiful body you maintain and you enjoy taking care of it.

You **begin to move** about the room, feeling how light you are. You are enjoying having full mastery of your body. Breathing deeply as you move, you easily maintain your optimum weight. Your body naturally responds to your care-taking. You now have the ability to partake in all of life. You can do all the things that once felt beyond you because of the cloak you were wearing. Without that heavy, cumbersome cloak, you have more freedom and energy than you ever thought possible. You exude youth and vitality. You have the energy to make your life better every day because you can now get on with it.

You naturally regulate your weight and there is no longer a battle with the scales. You are free to focus on making your life what you want it to be, feeling proud and confident in your body. You **look back and notice that cloak** lying on the floor. You recognize that it was never your enemy as you had thought. It was there to protect you when you needed it.

You now are able to take care of yourself and no longer need the cloak for protection. You **say goodby to the cloak** forever. Standing back in front of the mirror you feel completely safe and secure and wonderful about your beautiful body. Your inner beauty radiates to the world through your eyes and skin. You take good care of yourself in all ways and you now give yourself the kind, gentle treatment you give to others.

Every day the process of maintaining your optimum weight gets easier. You are drawn to those foods which produce radiant health and vitality. You want to take care of yourself in all ways and you give yourself time in each day to do so. This enables you to bring a healthier person to those you care for. It all begins with your love and care for yourself.

It is time now to return from your journey within. As you breathe, bring yourself back to a normal state of awareness. Each time you do this exercise, you bring this visualization closer to the reality of everyday life. You notice yourself doing things willingly which help you to reach your desired goals. You take time every day to perform this exercise in your process of creating the body you want.

Two-Level Healing

To be complete, healing must occur on two levels. You heal the mind and you heal the body; they are a package deal.

Healing the mind means releasing old hurts, beliefs and thought patterns from the past which are keeping you from making the most of your present.

Healing the body requires taking action to revitalize. This includes cleansing, affirming and meeting the needs of your body. Compulsive eating habits and fat simply melt away as your focus shifts from a sense of lack to a sense of fullness. As you complete this healing process, you are released from the past to live in what's happening now. You are free to find out who you are now, to enjoy being that fresh person and to become what you are able to be — healthy, slim and attractive.

Lynn And Ed And What They Saw

Lynn: The first person I went to for help told me to go home, look in the mirror and say 'I love you.' That was way too advanced for me then. Instead, one look and I broke into tears. I saw a woman slumping and sagging and weighed down, huddled inside all this fat. It made me want to go and eat something. I hated myself.

Ed: I looked pregnant — or, at least, like I had a watermelon between me and the world. My childhood wasn't all that bad but my parents weren't a bit interested in what I was up to. When they did try to change me, their approach was to put me down. I figured if my family hurts me this much, the people outside in the world will hurt me even more. I made sure people didn't get close enough to disappoint me. Sometimes you can't face even the chance that you're right.

An Affirmation To Stop Compulsive Eating
And Start Healthy Living

I release any blocks I may have to optimum health and well-being. I no longer hide behind my body to protect myself. I cope with my life directly and release the need for food or fat to serve this purpose. It is now safe for me to have a slim, fit body.

FIVE

Releasing Your Blocks: Body Remodeling Tools

 • The potential of watchful breathing.
• Detoxing our bodies.
• Affirmative walking.
• Power-centering with yoga.
• Imaging enthusiasm for exercising.

These are just a few of the areas of interest we can add to our new agenda as we grab hold of what we deserve: a life grounded in today, not smothered in pounds from the past.

Our capacity to give physical support to our psychological turning-around grows each time we say *No!* to the tyranny of our ancient response patterns. It's not just theory that the mind can either energize or devitalize the body, and the reverse is true, too. Changes in what you are doing with your body can affect your spirits, which in turn can give you more energy to help out your body. So when we are looking at permanent weight loss, we are looking at the total person — not just a waistline.

As we contemplate getting physical with one or more of the body events we will be describing, we may have to call on our Inner Parent to help us weather any natural resistance that may come after our initial excitement subsides. We all have a well-worn groove running through our psyches and sometimes slipping into its familiar ways feels good only because it is easy and known. We imagine the new and uncertain to be complicating our lives; we actually may long for the familiarity of the bad but known. So our Inner Parent may need to be enlisted to give us gentle support.

Try visualizing this Inner Parent as you at your most confident time in life. Experiment with calling on it regularly every time your Child feels tempted. If we backslide, it will not chastise us but, with compassion, let us find our own way, in our own time, away from that negative coping which has become mechanical and harmful and toward that which is humane and happy.

Let what was, stay in the past. Let what is, be now.

Breathing In Health

The power of our breath to heal our bodies is greatly underestimated by many. I was a confirmed skeptic until, in the spirit of nothing-lost experimentation, I discovered this age-old truism for myself.

For some time I had been aware of a need to clear negativity from my body, to revitalize. I was young but felt old, with zero stamina. Cobwebs seemed to be clogging my lungs.

Rebirthing was recommended to me by a colleague. I laughed and said "Re-what? That sounds ridiculous."

I tried it, anyway, of course. It was time to experiment with the unknown since the known — the old ways of coping — were part of the problem. To my amazement and relief, it was simply a series of guided breathing sessions which, indeed, had a profound effect on my body.

One rebirther, Suzanne Ponath in Dallas showed me how much I had underestimated what could be done with the breath. I found my body springing to life. I felt less fatigued. My compulsive eating subsided. Old blocks were being released and my stress level was reduced. I had more energy and clarity than I had experienced in a very long time. It was as if 15 years had fallen away from my age.

A revitalized, healthy body does not tolerate excess food.

This breath work training affected my entire life and was especially helpful during exercise. I became able to relieve stress through simple breathing practices; previously this stress would have resulted in eating episodes. Where had my lungs been all my life? What a tool for change! Today, rebirthing classes are offered all over the country and books on breathing are readily available. For a fitness approach to learning breathing techniques, there is Ian Jackson's *The Breathplay Approach to Whole Life Fitness*, great for revitalizing the cells and creating power and energy in the body. The techniques he describes can be used while doing daily exercise routines. Working with your body, not against it, makes it your ally in the process of saying no to too much food.

If You Hate To Exercise

If, so far, you haven't been able to talk yourself into exercising as a way of life, you probably have body blocks. We are naturally physical creatures. Through observing children at play and many tribal peoples, this becomes evident. They love to be active, to play and run. Using their bodies is an integral part of living.

What is it, then, that happens to this instinctive drive for movement and activity, for feeling good, in many adults? How do children who were born naturally comfortable with their bodies learn to reject them and find it difficult to keep them active?

In my experience of working with compulsive eaters and those who are overweight, I have seen a consistent pattern. Many have come from unhappy families which were alcoholic or dysfunctional in other ways. People with this background are known for living remote from their bodies. Physical abuse, blows, angry words and emotional pain are stored as body blocks and these, in turn, inhibit the ability to freely exercise and play. They depress the entire physical and emotional system.

If you have body blocks from your past, you probably feel a lack of energy and no motivation for exercise. You know you *should* exercise, you berate yourself for regressing if you periodically try, but you just can't get your heart into it on a permanent basis. Whenever you get started on any exercise program you lose motivation and quit. The energy is simply not available. You tell yourself it's because you're lazy and hate to exercise, but it may not be your fault. Chances are there are variables you are not consciously aware of that are sapping your energy and drive. These are the invisible limitations you may choose to clear from your body on your road to total well-being and aliveness.

Understanding and awareness are sometimes all you need to assist you in clearing these limitations from your life. Enlisting your Inner Parent to push gently but persistently may also help. Another way to overcome resistance is to give exercise a purpose beyond just physical activity.

Walking Away From Compulsive Eating

One exercise I have found colossally helpful is Affirmation Walking. You link your need to feed positives to your spirit with your body's need to move — what it was born to do.

To combine these two life-asserting activities, you may choose any affirmations from the chapter conclusions in this book or, especially, from the end of this chapter. Place these affirmations on tape and listen to them as you walk.

Affirmations may also be ordered on tape from the Institute for Personal and Professional Development (see Appendix for titles).

As you walk, breathe in deeply as you repeat the affirmations to yourself. On the out-breath, breathe out all negativity or resistance to health. It helps if you clothe these out-breaths in a symbolic color of grey or black. While walking, pull yourself erect and tall. Tighten your stomach, buttocks and legs on the out-breath.

Don't be too skeptical about the simplicity of this practice. The results can be amazing. The increased oxygen bathes all the cells and releases toxins stored in the body. It pumps vitality into your entire system. As a result of incomplete breathing and circulation, our bodies can age unnecessarily. This is the motivation for the megabucks some film stars pay for sessions in oxygen body tanks. Increasing the oxygen to the bloodstream enlivens the body, sharpens mental capacities and decreases depression in the system. I have found that doing these exercises while walking gives me the energy not only to stay with it but to extend my walking destinations.

Another technique I have found to be astoundingly effective is to imagine breathing in white, healing, cleansing light through the top of my head or through my mouth while walking. This can soothe the entire system, melt away worries and help you to feel vital and energetic.

Yo, Yoga!

The soundless, sweatless, weight-loss-enhancing exercise that can be done in the space of a towel: that's yoga!

It would be hard to find anyone who ever tried yoga (we're talking about the simplified forms, nothing fancy) who didn't love the way it made the body feel. In its purest form a transforming way of life, it is so potent that the smallest chips taken from it still are crammed with powerful benefits.

Today, you can find yoga packaged by Western teachers and writers for teens, grandmothers, athletes, etc. Yoga is superb for those who struggle with compulsive eating and fat. Its gentle movements (forget the lotus position and anything else that hurts or has to be forced — that's not real yoga, anyway) are subtly powerful and can contribute more to slimming you down than you might think. They also can be used to clear body blocks. There are good books available today for beginners. Adult education and independent studio classes abound, full of people of all shapes and ages. Yoga is A-1 for reducing built-up stress in the body and creating a deep sense of relaxation. Compulsive eaters need new ways to relax since stress reduction is often the purpose their eating has served.

Yoga also helps to create a centered feeling in the body. What's "centered?" Centering is what we need when we're not sure where we end and others begin. It's what we need when we're strung out or at loose ends. It's a good sense to refer to when we tend to hand over power to circumstances or food.

Whatever form of movement you choose, some sort of exercise — daily, therapeutic movement — is crucial for ridding yourself of compulsive eating and fat. There's no getting around it. When your body and mind have become convinced that now, for you, there has become no other option but to live a better life, they will stop resisting and start enjoying this new manifestation of the way they are valued.

A Visualization To Promote Exercising

To help reprogram the department of your mind that says *no* to exercise, a positive visualization can be very strengthening. To get the most from it, perform this mind exercise once a day for 30 days. It is designed to help you increase your metabolism and your desire for exercise.

Begin by sitting or lying in a comfortable position in a place where there are no distractions. Close your eyes and relax.

Imagine that relaxing energy is entering your body through the top of your head. As this energy passes through each part of your body, you feel the muscles loosen as all the tension is released. Begin to feel your scalp and forehead relax. Feel your eyes yield to this calming energy. Relax your cheeks, your mouth and your jaw. Let the tension leave your neck, slide off your shoulders, down your arms and out your hands.

Feel your chest relaxing, your stomach and back. Let the muscles in your hips relax. Relax your pelvic area, your thighs and legs all the way down to your toes. Let the relaxing energy flow through your body, allowing you to feel completely calm and comfortable.

Now, **imagine yourself in a natural setting** that is special to you. This is your corner of the universe where you can be alone, feeling safe and secure. You notice the beautiful colors and smell the rich aromas. You feel perfectly at ease, with a heightened sense of well-being. In this place you have the ability to completely focus your mind and create the reality you want for yourself. With every breath you feel light, soothing energy circulating throughout your body. As you breathe, **begin to shift your attention to your body.** Visualize the fat cells within your body. See these cells as small balloon-like structures under your skin which contain the fuel you've been carrying around with you. This fuel can be burned off to give you the energy you need in order to accomplish your goals.

See these balloon-like structures as having lids on them. As you continue to breathe, oxygen travels through your bloodstream and into the tissues of your body. The oxygen surrounds these fat cells and begins knocking off the lids as it releases the fuel into your system. Your metabolism now can burn off the fat and give you the energy to stay active.

Picture your metabolism as an engine that is turned on. Notice: Is it sluggish or does it run smoothly and burn fuel easily? At first, you may see this engine as sluggish. This may have impacted your ability to burn off stored fuel. Now, visualize this engine again, only this time see it heating up and running smoothly, with the ability to easily burn off excess fat. It may help you to picture this fat or fuel as gas in an automobile engine and to see your physical body as the body of the car. **Choose a body style that is sleek and elegant** with a bright, shining finish. Your metabolism is the engine in your automobile.

Visualize yourself again in a beautiful place. This time see yourself as this beautiful automobile with the road stretched out in front of you. You are filled with newness and excitement. You are traveling down this road with the pick-up of a brand new car. Everything is perfectly tuned, there is no excess baggage and you are designed for quick get-up-and-go. As you move, you enjoy the freedom and notice how good it feels to have energy and to feel the wind. You tune in to the excitement of this trip. You have the confidence and mobility to take part in all of life. You take pride in your body and you keep it bright and shiny.

Return your focus to the inner workings of your engine. Do a quick check of how it is running. If you detect any drag in your engine, mentally fix it so that you are running at your full capacity. Feel the exhilaration and excitement of sensing all your parts working together in harmony. You no longer need to store fuel. You keep your engine in excellent running condition. You keep it cleaned out so that there is no excess weight holding you back. **Notice how good it feels to have the power to enjoy life.** Look for opportunities to move and stay active. You are proud of your body and you keep it in fine shape.

Caring for yourself has become in all ways an essential part of your life. The benefits of this are so great that you look forward to the time of care-taking with excitement and enthusiasm. You easily maintain a lean, clean running machine. Taking care of yourself is now a natural part of your daily routine.

It is time, now, to leave this vision and **return to your normal awareness.** Every time you do this exercise you feel your body increasing its functioning and overall health. You also bring more energy, pride and enthusiasm into your everyday life. You enjoy taking care of yourself and keeping yourself physically fit and healthy. As you bring yourself back to normal awareness, you may drift off to sleep, knowing that these visions and feelings have been received at a deep level within your being.

Remember to repeat this exercise regularly in order to imprint your learning and reprogram your response center with positivity.

Get An Owner's Manual

Our car came with one — why not ourselves?

We may not like to acknowledge it at all but there's a lot about us that's mechanical as well as personal and just won't stand up under our sometimes-emotional approach to self-maintenance. On the other hand, to make matters a bit confusing, some human body machines are incredibly resilient. They take tremendous abuse before calling time-out. Many of us have family stories about a great-aunt or indestructible granddad who smoked six packs a day, ate six eggs and a half-pound of bacon for breakfast since time began and was finally dispatched to his or her heavenly reward in an accident on the skidway of a toboggan run at the age of 103. Believe it — they are the rare exceptions.

Mother Nature doesn't like to be taken lightly. In any journey toward health and happiness, the body figures centrally. It is an integral part and shouldn't be dared to withstand abuse. Take advantage of the wealth of publications available on tuning up your body and maintaining it in good condition. Your mind will thank your body many years from now. The wisdom you will have accumulated deserves to be housed in a body that lets you enjoy the new life you've created.

Imbalances in our diets and imbalances in our emotions ricochet off body and mind. It is well known that certain vitamin deficiencies can cause depression and fatigue. Compulsive eaters tend to favor certain food groups and ignore or minimize others. Some people are addicted to corn and wheat, for example, and for them, these foods, in turn, create more cravings. Imbalanced blood sugar levels in the body can influence fatigue and cravings. It is wise to check out the latest information on nutrition and perhaps investigate the use of vitamin and mineral supplements. Having your body's nutrient levels determined by a registered dietitian is often very valuable.

Could you be physiologically addicted to a certain food type? Maybe, if for no apparent reason you crave a particular food every day. You're not upset or worried and yet you want to eat. If you've been eating sugar daily, you're probably physiologically as well as emotionally addicted. It's amazing, but true, that recovery from sugar addiction can mimic the similar stages of more serious addictions which are not as socially acceptable. If you're really motivated, you teach yourself to outlast the craving and get support from others. You practice nurturing yourself in healthier ways each day.

Reprogramming your psychological and physiological appetites is not child's play. A graph charting most people's achievements and relapses for the first year would look like a buggy ride across the Rocky Mountains. But that makes the taste of success even sweeter.

Suzanne

Right now, my husband probably is walking around the block, thinking about what he can eat because of his exercising, that I can't. He walks 4.2 miles a day now . . . that's four times around. We used to walk together and it was a time we could talk. But then he quit because he didn't think slowing down to my leisurely pace was doing him much good.

Then he started again, walking faster, and I had to tell him that my body couldn't handle it, even though it wasn't even speed walking. My body would just tense up. But what happened with him, at the new speed his blood pressure has dropped dramatically. It finally clicked for him that real exercise makes you feel great. He comes home high, and he's 58. Meanwhile, I'm feeling rotten. I'll be 50 this year, and unless I get with some real exercise pretty soon, my life will have no quality. I belong to a health club now, but sometimes just thinking about having to stop everything to drive over and back every morning makes me not go. If only I could afford a home gym.

An Affirmation To Stop Compulsive Eating And Start Healthy Living

I recognize and release all self-defeating thought processes concerning exercise. I love my body and let go of the need to hurt it through carrying excess weight. I now visualize the fat on my body as stored energy and I create opportunities throughout each day to burn it off. I respond to my muscles' yearning for exercise.

I enjoy taking the time every day to release stress through stretching, deep breathing and movement. My body is my vehicle through life and I make sure to keep it in good condition. Here, inside, I have all the strength and willpower I need to achieve vibrant health.

SIX

"I'm So Angry, I Could . . . Eat!"

Of all the emotions compulsive eaters typically wrestle with, anger is at the top of the list as toughest to handle.

Or perhaps we should say it's the easiest to handle because usually, when it arises, it is quickly ticked off as no-win. Then it's deep-sixed. What is hardest to deal with are the inevitable repercussions on body and mind of this unnatural processing. Remember, there's no fooling Mother Nature. Her job is to record the tension and constriction in your body and do her best to compensate. Often, the task has become too big for any body to handle.

Anger is a feeling that can be frightening. If we express it, what will happen? Here's an example of the type of interaction and reaction many compulsive eaters experience.

Let's say we're married and our spouse leaves a pile of clothes on the bedroom floor. We get angry. We don't give ourselves permission to express it directly to the offender, so we discount our feelings and the problem. We see the noxious items and begin a slow burn. A warning flag goes up: beware of self-expression. Soon we decide to choose one of the following options in dealing with the situation:

1. Discount the significance of it. We tell ourselves, "It isn't important enough to argue about. It really isn't that big a deal."
2. We discount the solvability. Our thoughts are, "It won't do any good to talk about it anyway. It goes in one ear and out the other. There's just no caring about my preferences."
3. We discount ourselves or the person with "Slobs stay slobs" or "I shouldn't complain. After a day's hard work, I guess it's to be expected. I'm just being petty."

The Quiet Rage Within

Openly, we don't say anything. We pick up the mess. As we do, some of us bend over backwards in a psychological loop-the-loop. We deny even further that there's a problem by being cordial to the offender — after an ominous silence draws the person's attention.

Our spouse notices we're "not ourself" and says, "What's the matter?"

"Nothing," we say in a small voice with a Mother Teresa smile.

Something is obviously wrong, someone is obviously angry, but no one is enthusiastic about a confrontation. Dishonesty is the welcome alternative.

The miscreant walks away and we're left with suppression and agitated feelings bubbling to the surface that demand soothing.

We replay in our heads several dozen dialogs we would like to have had with our spouse but didn't dare. If we just have to talk to someone, we ventilate the most intolerable of our frustrations over the situation to our best friends. But, usually, the residue of unresolved emotions is oppressive. Not only are we still stuck with the original anger over the situation but layered on top of that is the further resentment that we can't express ourselves without dire repercussions.

Now let's see, what could we do next that would comfort us . . .?

This suppressed anger often is the root of compulsions and addictions. Each unresolved incident is added to a pile of similar experiences whose growing size, in itself, results in more quiet raging within. Then you eat and — magic! — you don't feel as angry any more. You've been able to do something to yourself that feels good. Food is your sedative. It helps calm you down and appeases the angry beast you wish did not dwell within.

It's only a temporary appeasement, though. That "beast" in you actually is a lady named Justice. She knows that you deserve your say, without being punished for having an opinion.

According to several research reports, over 70 percent of the compulsive eaters surveyed reported feeling calm, tired, sleepy, sluggish, lazy or groggy after a compulsive eating episode. They were convinced that they found relief from frustration, anger and anxiety in eating, although none recognized sedation as the goal (see Chart 1, The Anger Trap).

For many people I've talked with, the amount of weight on their bodies is the symbol for how much anger they've stuffed or trapped inside.

Suppressed Anger As Illness

Repeated gunnysacking or suppressing anger eventually leads to depression and incapacitation. It may result in a dependence on sedatives. There's so much emotion that has collected, so many "little things" that have built up. These feelings become generalized and you are rather unsuccessful at putting them into words. You're afraid that if you talked you might "explode." Or, perhaps, you are exploding at minor annoyances as an inappropriate

Passivity

Inside-yourself you	External you
1. Discount the problem/feeling. (Ignore it, act as though it doesn't exist or you don't feel it.)	1. Do nothing, take no action.
2. Discount the significance of the problem. ("That wasn't important enough to bring up.")	2. Compensate by smiling and acting as though there's no problem
3. Discount the solvability. ("It won't do any good, anyway, to bring it up.")	3. Become angry or irritated inside and you — eat, drink, smoke, fight, kick your foot, etc.
4. Discount yourself or others. ("Who am I to say anything? They don't deserve to know.")	4. Get depressed and say, "I don't know what is the matter. I'm just depressed." Result is illness, headaches, obesity, ulcers, compulsive eating, drinking or smoking.

The ultimate form of passivity
is movement toward death

Chart 1. The Anger Trap

way to ventilate major unspeakable transgressions on the part of people important to you.

The final stage of suppression is illness. You may have ulcers, irritable bowel syndrome, chronic headaches, extreme depression, trouble with reproductive organs or obesity. Many of the people I have seen in my practice have had major surgery or illness. All were very angry people and did not know how to express their anger. All the resentment they had carried toward someone else — mother, father or spouse, usually — was making them ill.

Tilt! Your Life Is Off-Balance

Compulsive eating and being overweight are signs that your life is suffering from imbalance. Something isn't quite right. It's your body's way of telling you that you must make some changes or suffer some consequences potentially as awful as those you have been eating to avoid.

Excessive eating and obesity are uncomfortable, limiting and expensive states to maintain. They never result simply because "I like to eat" or "I just love food." Although these statements may be quite true in themselves, they hold as well for many people without eating disorders. With a healthy appetite, natural internal mechanisms kick in when you've had enough to satisfy your biological needs.

Our bodies instinctively move toward health — when our heads aren't holding them back.

Children regulate their food intake naturally if they haven't learned to disregard body signals as a result of years of unhealthy training. If you generally keep on swallowing to the point of being painfully full or if you eat excessive snacks when your body isn't hungry, then you, too, have been taught to disregard the messages your body is giving you.

The inability to express anger may be something that you can identify in yourself. If so, losing weight and kicking the habit of compulsive eating also means learning how to express anger. You can't lose the weight and ignore the drive to self-express. If you do that, your body will find a way such as heart disease or ulcers to manifest distress for you. Suppressed anger is a time bomb. Take it seriously and detonate it before it erupts in an unhealthy way. Feelings are natural and healthy; suppression and denial are potentially life-threatening.

Martyrdom Is An Unnatural Act

Anger is often a result of feeling that others have taken advantage of you. But consider: Maybe we have expected a level of sensitivity from people that actually borders on clairvoyance. Our *yes*es sound as though we mean them.

Many compulsive eaters were never taught how to say *no*, especially a caring *no*. But being straightforward when we're too tired or too harassed to help is a natural, democratic action. When we don't treat ourselves as kindly as we treat others, we see our emotions and our bodies rebelling, no matter how our minds want them to behave. Then we are of less use to other people and we become lax custodians of our own bodies and lives.

When we have created a disharmony, a dis-ease in our own environment, we suffer for the unnatural strain we assumed we should somehow be able to manage. This isn't to say we should never overextend ourselves, no matter what. We can get away with it once in a while, but there are some burdens we can't shoulder even if we want to and even if others could. You don't have to admire your own limitations to respect the incontestable fact that all humans are limited in different ways at different times. Anyone who thinks you're an exception would benefit from hearing that all mankind is not born equal. Saints are not the norm; being regarded a sinner is not the alternative.

Maybe we learned it was better to give than to receive, so we say *yes* to many things people ask us to do that we really don't want to do? We volunteer for activities, taking on more than our share at home, church or work. Somebody wants us to babysit and we say *yes*. Someone else wants us to bake the cookies for Scouts and we say, "Okay, I'll do that, too." Our boss overloads us with work and we say "Yes, I'll have time." We either don't really want to do it or we just can't.

We may not know how to set limits for ourselves. We find we're running 60 to 80 hours a week. We may work 40 hours on a job, come home to clean and cook and yet never demand support after we see there is some disinterest in helping. We try to do all the things people want us to do. Naturally, we feel resentful later. Nobody studied our lives to see if we were overloaded when we so kindly agreed to be dumped on even further. Whenever you consider a firm *no*, you feel so guilty that you quickly rule it out.

When you feel resentful and petty, you don't dare tell anyone what's going on. It's too embarrassing. "They should know!" you silently scream into the refrigerator, where once again you have gone for comfort.

Being What You Are

Learning how to express anger is essential to breaking away from compulsive eating. No longer can we allow ourselves to believe that we have no right to be angry — or "I shouldn't be feeling this way and no one wants to hear about it."

Instead of allowing the Critical Parent inside to tell you how you should or shouldn't be, be natural! You really have no choice if you want to be healthy.

If you're angry, you're angry. If you are angry over something another person considers petty, acknowledge that EVERYONE needs the freedom to get angry sometimes over petty as well as major issues. It's okay to say to someone, "I don't always need to be understood. I don't always need to understand you, either. But sometimes I do need to be allowed to let off steam!"

When we don't communicate our feelings straightfor-
wardly to family, friends and co-workers, they get a different impression of who we are. When our true feelings
become apparent — as they always do, in one way or
another — then we're broadcasting mixed messages, causing angry misunderstandings that explanations aren't likely to make right.

Fortunately, today many books are available on improv-
ing your personal communcation skills so that you don't
lose people worth having in your life. There may be, of
course, some people so troubled themselves that honest
communication is impossible. It's up to you to decide if you
want to sacrifice your health and happiness to their needs.

When you form the habit of giving yourself permission
to express your emotions and work things out with Significant Others, you will find a decrease in the urge to
eat. Refer to Chart 2 to reinforce your new approach to
releasing anger. Take advantage of all the resources in the
health community where you live. Don't let your latent
anger continue to work as that time bomb, making you its
primary victim when it explodes.

Learned Passivity Begins At Home

If you feel uncomfortable expressing anger, you probably learned passivity in one of two types of families:

Type S (for *saintly*) or C (for *cool*): families in which no
anger is expressed at all, or in which children were not
allowed to express it, ever. Perhaps anger simmered but
you learned early that it is not okay to be angry. You
probably received the message that you couldn't be a good
person, or a good Christian, and show anger. Maybe your
family considered emotionality "not cool" or a character-
istic of the "common herd."

Type R (for *raging*): This family has a hair-trigger tem-
per, is full of excessive anger. You may have learned your
fear of anger in this violent family where anger meant
pain and aggression and you were often the victim.

A safer way to express, rather than suppress, anger:

1. Identify what you are feeling.

Anger	Hurt
Fear	Jealousy
Sadness	Other _____

2. Choose resolution instead of "gunnysacking."

3. List options for resolution.

Confront
Forgive

4. Take action.

Chart 2. Springing The Anger Trap

Families are amazingly influential. Now, as adults, we know that there are many kinds of fathers and many kinds of mothers. They have conflicting philosophies about how their families should be dealt with, how their children should be raised. We know parents can even disagree about the various merits or demerits of a child. Nevertheless, we took their idiosyncratic opinions very seriously for years as children. Perhaps because of the mystique of birth and lifegiving, most of us still give those early opinions some degree of weight. Whether they're positive or negative, they came from those special people, our own parents.

In learning to deal with anger in a way that does not drive us into the kitchen, we can consider how we were shaped psychologically as children and see if this is an area where we can renew ourselves. Maybe we don't have to react any longer from the dysfunctional past. A better understanding of our beginnings can help us become more authentically ourselves, more realistically expressive and less "hungry" for a satisfying life, now being created.

Cindy

When I was a kid, I was a terrific swimmer, so my dad insisted I join the swim team at school. I hated it. I hated competing. But he wouldn't hear any of that. Just called me lazy. So before any swim event I would eat a whole box of cookies and drink two cartons of chocolate milk. I remember feeling fat and the coaches telling me that I *was* getting fat. When we'd all line up on the edge of the pool, I really stood out and people would make fun.

So I started losing weight. Eventually, I couldn't find clothes small enough for me. I could feel my backbone when I sat down, I became so thin. When I told my father I wanted to drop off the team, he flew into a rage and said sitting around would only make me get fat again. I quit and did gain. Since then, I've always had weight problems. I'd really like to get rid of this fat for good, sign up for group therapy, get into another exercise class, but my husband just laughs. He doesn't take me seriously. And he's the one with the money.

An Affirmation To Stop Compulsive Eating And Start Healthy Living

I give myself permission to express myself, my feelings and desires. It's okay for me to have what I want and to feel what I feel. I no longer squelch myself with food or fat. I have patience with myself and others. I accept myself where I am today. I surround myself with people who accept my humanness as I accept theirs. I am a friend to myself.

SEVEN

Eating To Say No: Weight As A Sexual Turn-Off

True or false: Human beings, with their potential for strong sexual needs, their hidden agendas, their sometimes misleading friendliness, their hangups, their unpredictable fickleness, their ability to gain your confidence, then wound deeply, aren't as hard to handle as — potato chips!

Letting food run interference in the arena of relationships is a familiar theme among compulsive eaters. If the pounds are really allowed to pile up, we may find ourselves sidelined, largely out of the game. But that's okay with us. We'd rather stay home, anyway.

Fat and food can become vital to coping with a variety of attitudes stemming from childhood experiences that relate to sexuality. Some people who feel they have absolutely no control over food also feel that way about relationships in general or, specifically, with members of the opposite sex. Some of the fear-connections involving fat and husbands, wives or boyfriends, include:

- Becoming attractive to potential sexual partners out-side the marriage or primary relationship.
- Losing overeating as a shared form of entertainment.
- Being mistaken as a promiscuous woman with an attractive figure.
- Actually turning into a promiscuous woman if weight is lost.
- "Inviting" a rerun of a childhood nightmare — sexual abuse.

Drawing Boundaries With Fat

Our boundaries are where others end and we begin. They mark the areas where we have to say *no*, instead of *yes*. The inability to set boundaries can lead to compulsive eating and being overweight.

Many obese married women have watched their own mothers subjugate major needs to their husbands and children. They had never been taught by example how to take care of themselves first, or *why* they should take care of themselves first. As they lived lives of quiet despera-tion, many were seldom heard to complain. Instead, their feelings were apparent in their dull eyes and were demon-strated in quiet, seething anger. Any time they tried to define their space or care for themselves, they were over-whelmed by guilt. Anger and guilt: prime ingredients in a recipe for compulsive eating.

A Form Of Prostitution

The pattern of self-sacrifice for their men is so in-grained in the fiber of their being that some women are completely out of touch with their own needs. They feel compelled to give themselves totally to their husbands, an inclination their husbands support wholeheartedly, as a rule. This sounds either noble or necessary to their mar-riage for these women and it may have Mother's tacit seal of approval. But because it is so lopsided and the negative effects so obvious, we know this attitude is not harmonious with who they really are.

If a lifestyle continues to produce negative results for years, then we can suspect we are choosing it because:

1. We think it's giving us something we can't get any other way.
2. We deserve it, it's simply the way our lives have to be.
3. We don't understand how we got into it and we doubt we have the energy or ability to get out of it.

Wrong, on all counts — if we really want change. Understanding is the bridge from nowhere to somewhere.

Seductive Lifestyles

A malfunctioning lifestyle may not look seductive on the surface but it can be full of built-in traps. Just the time and effort invested in it may make many women hang in there. They have never focused on building anything for themselves. When young, they were never shown or told they should or could be a role model. Later, the time never seemed to be right or available for self-expression or self-fulfillment.

For so long they've felt powerless to change. Time has turned what began as a feeling that they weren't too effective into a mountain of conviction that self-help wouldn't work for them.

An exploration of the conclusions we drew about childhood events and an understanding of the way we buried the incomprehensible hurts we couldn't deal with, are just the dynamite we need to blast these negative opinions out of our way.

A Man's Problem, Too

Women aren't the only ones who can use excess weight to draw boundaries with the opposite sex. Gregg, a state park ranger, at one time had weighed over 400 pounds. He lost weight and shortly thereafter was married. He became very unhappy in this marriage and eventually filed for divorce. After the divorce, back came 100 more pounds. It made him a safe friend for women, he said. He no longer had to worry about marriage or sexual involvement.

To spring this trap, it is necessary to deal with and release fears of the opposite sex. This may include taking care of "unfinished business" with Mom or Dad. It is also crucial to realize that you don't have to use fat to say *no* for you. You can learn to set limits and boundaries for yourself in a way that enhances your emotional and physical health. Allow yourself to experiment and to explore.

Wanton Woman Wanting Out

In therapy and in seminars on compulsive eating, I have seen a number of women whose appearance was matronly but who make stunning statements like, "If I lose this weight I'm afraid I will go out and have an affair." Often their spouses do not fulfill them and the repressed role they've assumed covers up a naturally frustrated female. They are so repressed that they actually believe they might rage out of control with sexuality, given a body of normal weight.

Lila, a 36-year-old travel agent, was radically opposed to society's emphasis on *svelte* as the standard of beauty. Yet when I asked her to complete the sentence, *Now that I'm married, I can't look thin because* . . . she shifted uncomfortably in her chair and responded with arch-conservatism:

"Married women shouldn't be sexy to other men . . . I don't want other men to be attracted to me because I have to turn away from temptation . . . because I feel guilty when I fantasize . . . because now that I'm married I'm supposed to look matronly . . . because if I look matronly, it shows that I'm happy and taken."

To my sentence, *If I'm married, slender and sexy, then I must be . . .*, she thoughtfully added, ". . . on the prowl because happily married people don't have to stay thin and sexy . . ."

Compulsive eating can be an expensive form of divorce insurance. Understanding ourselves is a better policy.

Weight is often a way to remain loyal to a spouse who does not otherwise merit it. Many women fear they will have to divorce their husbands if they lose weight or stop eating compulsively. The weight and lethargy resulting from compulsive eating become the shackles that control that wanton woman suspected of lurking inside.

Lila eventually released all of this, was able to let go of her prejudices against achieving a healthy weight after marriage, dropped many pounds and neither defended nor denied the extra weight she still continued to carry. She was happy in the body she had created and able to accept further loss when she was ready.

Not Me, I'm Spiritual

Our society teaches certain values associated with being a "spiritual" person. The church can become another parent, giving equally powerful messages, both positive and negative. Distorted church indoctrination can have a very negative effect, feeding into doubts already present, when it departs from teaching self-love and goodness and instead emphasizes original badness. The implications to many are clear: Sex is too exploitative and selfish to be part of the goodness taught as an ideal. To women who take this to heart, the effects can be devastating, reinforcing their existing doubts.

An integration of sexuality with a feeling of being good is needed here. To slim the body and get into shape, you must first believe that you can have a healthy looking body and still be good and moral.

Fat is not any more spiritual than thin — although carrying it around may get you to heaven much sooner.

Fat As Protector From Violent Crime

Sexual trauma — rape or incest — creates within its many victims the fear of ever again being attractive. If women with this trauma in their pasts still feel responsible for what happened to them, being fat may be their way to assure it can't happen again. It doesn't matter how long ago the crime occurred or how young they were at the time. The feeling of responsibility lingers and the victim may think, "I caused it, and it's not safe for me to be pretty."

The sense deep inside that their bodies are bad often lingers. Although the trauma may have happened as much as 20 years ago, some women seem to have caught and still carry the illness of the molester, including sexual confusion, shame and guilt. Adults with this history usually deprive themselves of closeness, believing that they are bad and do not deserve to be loved.

Casey, a woman in one of my compulsive eating groups, was a very attractive woman with large almond eyes and thick, shoulder-length black hair. She was 45 and had never been married. When she joined the group she was 45 pounds overweight but had been 150 pounds above her norm. She had just been through another diet program and was terrified that it would, again, be a waste of money and she would be gaining it back. She was eager to break the cycle.

In therapy she revealed that she had been molested by her grandfather from the age of nine through adolescence. She then started drinking and putting on weight. The only way she could have a physical relationship with a man was to become totally drunk. When these remembrances first came out, she laughed them off — another defense. Gradually she stopped laughing and cleansed herself, in therapy, from blame for his illness. Her entire demeanor changed. On one date at the beginning of therapy, her date said how attractive she was. She went home and ate chocolate all night long, gaining 20 pounds. By the end of therapy, compliments were no longer a threat and she had successfully said *no* and *yes* without liquor.

Clearing An Incestor

A helpful exercise which will clear an incestor or negative body image is called the Purification Visualization.

Picture yourself in a pond or hot tub full of water. Or actually sit in your bathtub. See yourself as washing away all negativity, all impurities from your body. If you are in your tub, you can make a ritual of this by washing and cleansing all the parts of your body.

If you were molested or traumatized, see yourself washing away the illness of the violator. Talk to your body as you do this. Say to your arms, legs, breasts, genitalia, "You are good and I love and cherish you." Lovingly cleanse your body with as much tenderness as you would a baby. That's who you really have inside, you know. You still include that precious innocent child whose body needs to be treated with as much respect as a sacred temple.

Lean back and dip your head into the water. See all worries, fears and anxieties washing away. Cleanse and restore the purity, the feeling of essential goodness.

It may help to put white candles in the room with you. Turn out the lights and light the candles to set the mood. If you are so inclined, it may also feel good to see white light coming in through the top of your head, bringing life, clarity and purity to your whole system.

Breathe out any negativity from your mouth. Visualize this as black or grey mist as you exhale. You also may want to pray to God or to what you consider your Higher Power to help you clear any negativity and restore your body to its original vitality.

Be patient and gentle with yourself. Repeat the exercise as often as you need to, for as long as you need.

Joanne

My mother kind of gave the impression that she had to do everything that was hard and joyless. Like if it weren't for Dad and us kids, she could have had an interesting life.

Dad's message was basically that life is hard, you end up doing an awful lot of things you don't want to do and you get trapped. You have no choice.

About each other? Well, Mom made it fairly clear that men were babies, can't do anything for themselves, or they could be selfish, inconsiderate brutes. I would be just as happy if I could do without them.

The message from Dad about women was that women are emotional, illogical and just plain crazy. But they have a definite place, subservient to men. I mean, he didn't say that in so many words but it was pretty clear. It was like 'I love your mother but you don't get what you need from women.'

Mainly I figured it was like giving up your soul to be married. When I really started eating, in my early 20s, my mother complained, of all things, that I wouldn't get a man, and my father let me know that it was disappointing to have a fat daughter. Like I was less of a woman all around.

So I'm 39 and have my soul and no ring.

An Affirmation To Stop Compulsive Eating And Start Healthy Living

I release the need to hide my body with fat. I no longer need fat to protect me from intimacy. My inner qualities don't change with my outer appearance. I accept all of myself. As my own friend, I choose not to hurt or injure myself in any way. I do things to make myself happy. It is time for me to actualize my potential.

EIGHT

Fear, Families And Fat

 Family dynamics — what makes a family tick — frequently are at the root of lifelong eating disorders.

- If you have come from a family of big eaters where everyone is overweight, then you are likely to be ridiculed or ostracized if you make a move toward being slim.
- If your family pressured you as a child to lose weight, compulsive eating may have become your message to be left alone.
- If Mom fed or continues to feed your emotional needs with fattening food, you still may be accepting that form of nourishment into your 30s, 40s and 50s-plus.

Unresolved grief, abandonment, poverty, criticism, a host of siblings competing for food — all these issues and more — stemming from experiences not clearly understood as a child can make eating in a healthy way very problematical as an adult.

Some people, of course, have to deal with more emotional baggage coming from the past than others. There are lives that are very complicated, in which many concerns and confusions have to be unraveled. In the stories to follow of former compulsive eaters who have disentangled themselves from leftover family problems, you may see a part of yourself.

Dictionaries define *compulsive* as an irresistible, repeated and irrational impulse to do something. *Irrational* is simply lacking the power to reason, which describes the undeveloped minds of all children. Now that you have the capacity to understand as an adult, you can explore your memory of those bewildering situations you found yourself in as a child and see what they were all about. You can move past the child's decision to bury what was not understandable. You can venture beyond the hurt because you acknowledge that, as an adult, you are now empowered with the ability to reason. The more motivated you are to use that reason and dump the past, the less you are able to eat irrationally. You lose the ability to be a compulsive eater without diets and sophisticated weight-loss programs.

Staying Familiar To Family

Compulsive eating and staying overweight are sometimes essential to belonging. If you have come from a family of big eaters where everyone is overweight, then you are likely to be ridiculed or ostracized if you are slim. You may have unwritten Family Membership Rules. If you observe family units in which staying in shape is valued, you'll see that in these families with high self-esteem, it's okay for everyone to look good, feel good and seek fulfillment.

In families with lower self-esteem, there may be alcoholism, compulsive eating, obesity, depression or chronic illness. To be accepted, you must be sick, fat or miserable like everyone else. If not, you're seen as "uppity" or "too good" for the rest of the family. You actually may be told, "You think you're better than anyone else." This is very powerful and very subtle in its effect. The bottom line is, "If you want us to love you, you have to have the same problems we have. Then we can be comfortable around you."

When compulsive eating becomes your message to parents to leave you alone, it may reflect your assertion that they had no right to pressure you to change. We can become very stuck in these family dynamics, never growing up because we have made our whole lives a statement of rebellion against one or two people. This is part of what is called "enmeshment." Enmeshment occurs when one is emotionally entangled with family. It can continue regardless of age or geographical distance from parents. Enmeshment ends with understanding.

Going Home For A Visit

Salina, a 36-year-old art sales consultant from a family of seven children, had struggled with extra pounds all her life. She had gone into therapy to recover her confidence after failing at a dozen diet programs. Now she had dropped 75 pounds and at 125 was looking good. Then she went home for Easter.

Opening her mom's freezer, she was overwhelmed by the stockpile inside: six boxes of donuts, eight cartons of ice cream, seven coffee cakes, fattening processed lunch meats and rolls galore. The refrigerator was bursting with breads, milk, cheese, pasta dishes and soft drinks. When she accompanied Mom to the grocery the next day (Mom grocery-shopped daily), she was floored when more packages of cookies landed in the cart, after their just having finished dozens the day before.

"Have mercy!" she begged Mom.

"But Jeannie wants some," Mom said. "No, Jeannie doesn't," said Salina. Her very overweight sister had complained the day before about too many snacks in the house.

Her mother replied, reaching for another bag of cookies, "Well, if you can't control your eating, that is your problem. You're just going to have to learn to!"

At home, seven brothers and sisters — all overweight except Salina — were standing in the kitchen before dinner. Some were grumbling about all the food available and finally one daughter said, "Ma, stop buying all this food!"

"But I only do it because I love you!" said the bewildered mother. It was obvious to all that (1) Mom had a problem with food and (2) she didn't know any other way to love.

In a flash, Salina saw the situation. Her mother had told her that if she didn't lose weight she wouldn't get a man and that, basically, that all that mattered in life. Paradoxically, Mom had so many adult daughters at home to keep her company because they were overweight and socially shy. In therapy, Salina was able to release her anger at her mom and stabilize her weight. She married at this time, also.

Mixed Messages From Mother

Volatile enmeshment issues are created when there are mixed messages passing from mothers to daughters. When a mother criticizes her daughter's weight frequently and at other times pushes fattening foods, the results may be devastating. A mixture of confusion, guilt and depression follow. It is very difficult for daughters from such relationships to marry and emotionally separate from their mothers. Many such women never marry. Those who do marry often have great difficulty in committing emotionally to their husbands.

In therapy, they come to realize that they are bound to their mothers in a subtle yet powerful way. They are subtly made to feel responsible for their mother's lives and happiness. Accompanying this is tremendous resentment. The relationship is riddled with conflict. Wherever they may live, they tend to "stay home" emotionally with Mom.

The breakthrough occurs when the daughter realizes that Mother wants her to be fat so she won't leave her mother at home to face the world alone. These women often are amazed when they realize that being fat has been their way of responding to their mothers' unconscious wishes. This can be the beginning of a lasting change in behavior.

Mama's Treasure Hunt

The controller of a medium-size construction company came to me at the age of 39 with 25 pounds he couldn't lose, panicky that he was going to develop a heart condition. All his compulsive eating was done between midnight and five in the morning, and much of it he didn't remember.

"Sometimes I'll recall slicing cheese very quietly," he said, "so no one would know I was up, but often I don't know I've eaten during the night — except if there's jam on my pajamas the next morning!"

He was a sleep-eater. It began when he was a little boy and was a sleepwalker. His mother, knowing this, would leave treats in the refrigerator and he would find them there in the middle of the night, sometimes consciously and sometimes not.

She would put happy little notes on the refrigerator like "Hi, hope you enjoy this treat!" It was great fun until, in adulthood, he couldn't shake the need for a nighttime foodfest. What started out as a cute way for Mama to love her baby boy became a pot belly and frustration. The middle-age treasure hunt felt good while it was happening but the consequences weren't as desirable. When he tried to eliminate food, he felt an emotional emptiness which took some effort to pinpoint.

She Giveth, She Taketh Away

I've known several women with weight problems who say they were skinny as children. Teena, a 29-year-old homemaker who lacked the confidence to get a job because of her weight, said she was known as "Boney Maroney" as a child.

"My mama would load me up with milk shakes, heavy breads and cakes and things to put weight on me," she said. "But once I had gained, she withheld all the goodies. It was feast or famine. I dreaded my weight getting back to normal because then the fun foods disappeared. I felt betrayed for doing what she wanted me to do."

As an adult, she was 125 pounds overweight and never without her favorite junk foods. Once she ate so much chocolate cake she "overdosed" and passed out. She regained control of her eating with a better understanding of her mother and herself.

"Positive" Family Messages About Fat

Janice was a gentle woman in her late 20s with a flawless, radiant complexion, deep green eyes and a talent for dressing with flair, even though she was 145 pounds overweight. She loved clothes. And she never had been on a date.

Like many people with a serious weight problem, she had not realized how many positive messages her family had been feeding her over the years about staying fat. We tried some sentence-completion exercises to bring out buried programming broadcast by her family. The sentence, *Warnings I heard involving weight loss were* . . . reminded her of such subtle messages as, "You shouldn't lose so much that, if you get sick, you don't have any more to lose." She recalled getting such impressions as, "You have to eat to live, to have a good time, to belong, to be a part of your family, to show appreciation, to kill time."

CAUTION: Surgeon General warns that families can be hazardous to your health!

With another technique called Gestalt therapy, Janice was encouraged to visualize her mother in a chair across from her and to begin a conversation with her in which she could be perfectly frank. In these dialogues she realized she was keeping her fat on her body so she wouldn't have to grow up emotionally and leave home. Yet she also was using it suicidally because she really was so immensely tired and bored with the way she was living, alone and without significant friends. She explored the ways in which she had been used as a buffer between her warring parents and the sense of feeling guilty because she was failing at this task, her only real purpose in life.

The pressures and fears she experienced whenever she considered leaving home had been placated with an excess of food that kept her obese and prevented her from making a change. "You'll always be our baby," her mother said, clinging to her throughout years of depressing marital discord. Janice thought her mother might very well die if she grew up.

Janice also tried a conversation with her fat in the Gestalt chair — which sounds amusing but, in fact, can result in a great deal of new awareness. Janice said to Fat:

"I'm afraid if I lose you I won't be as together. All the effort will be wasted. I'll never be satisfied with what I am. I'm afraid I won't have any rear end or hips and I am afraid I would hate my body anyway if I were slim."

Behind the problem are many years, many pounds, many issues, most of which lie out of psychological sight but must manifest somehow. That *somehow* is weight for compulsive eaters. Compulsive eaters often have a great deal of ambivalence about weight loss, and numerous unresolved personal problems are drawn into the chosen way of resolution — eating. Several fears not consciously recognized may be involved. For a serious drop in weight, food must be put in its place. The only permanent way to achieve this is to buckle down and deal determinedly with the source. Otherwise, any try at weight loss that skirts the core issues results in the emotional subconscious propelling the self back to eating, almost as if it were a life saver rather than a life destroyer. Meanwhile, the conscious mind is creating conflict with its *I don't want this weight, I don't want it!*

What did it take? Honesty, courage and a willingness to replace a new understanding for all those programmed notions that had kept her stuck. Plus a determination to stop being fed up with life.

Several months after leaving therapy, Janice called to say she was losing weight again. "I sort of relapsed a bit, but you prepared me for that and I was patient with myself. Now I've lost 50 more pounds. And I'm seeing so many more things about myself. I'm surprised that instead of making me feel badly, it's liberating. You can know you have problems but you feel helpless until you know why you're hanging on to them!"

Some of the realizations she valued included taking responsibility for herself or her life and that she was doing much better because she was starting that process of accepting where she truly was. She was happy that she was adapting to her changed understanding of her life — a vital point where 310 pounds are concerned because a good life depended on those pounds plunging.

Meaningful weight loss means major psychological adjustments. Letting go requires flexibility. Get in training now!

Swans Surviving As Fat Ducks

Some compulsive eaters I've talked to were faced with rejection as children for their attractiveness or talents in jealous families. Their solution to being trapped in these situations was to eat their way into a less enviable state. Often this is done unconsciously by a child too young to fully realize the problem but aware that standing out positively from the others in the family isn't going to help. By adulthood, the former child is ready to understand the coping techniques of human nature. One young woman, a typographer, said, "If I feel good about my life and body, I'll feel guilty about being happy because my mother never was."

Cases Of Neglect

Nancy's history included extreme abandonment and neglect. As an infant, she had been left in an attic, unattended, while her mother was hospitalized. She came close to starving to death. Her father found her — skinny, scared and covered with rashes from not being changed or cleaned. This left her with a deeply imbedded fear of not having her needs met and of not having enough.

At the age of 42, a successful real estate appraiser, she was still padding her body and her home to ward off the fear of starving or not having enough. "When I cleaned out my attic, for example, I noticed a light feeling inside, both physically and emotionally," she said. "Then, I started experiencing this paralyzing fear. I felt as though I were in a car with my feet on the accelerator and the brake at the same time."

Her dread of not having enough had fueled her eating compulsion for years. As she came to a new understanding of herself, she found she was able to release her grip on food and on possessions. A visualization that made a major difference with the latter problem began with imagining her home as her body. I suggested she view the excess stashed in different parts of her house as fat on her body. She was also to assign body parts to the different areas of her home. The most obvious example of this was her kitchen, seen as her stomach.

Next, she was asked to do a spring cleaning and to begin releasing the excess from her environment. She was to imagine the excess as fat released from her body, tossing out anything from her environment that supported her obesity.

When she started the exercise, she had a home that looked like an upscale flea market. Afterwards, the house lost weight as she did, becoming considerably lighter and brighter.

Another woman, Margaret, owner of an employment agency for temporary personnel, was raised in such poverty that she remembered eating ketchup sandwiches and the fat off meat to feel full. As a business executive, she enjoyed ordering full meals with big steaks that made her feel affluent, although poverty was no longer a possibility.

Reina, a 27-year-old accountant, nearly starved to death as an infant. For reasons unknown to her, ice cream was available in her childhood only when there were visitors. When she grew up, binging on ice cream warded off bouts of feeling deprived emotionally. After therapy, when she finally realized the source of what she was doing, she reported that she was unable to finish a serving of her old frozen friend.

Both women learned new ways of loving and nurturing their child from the past through gentleness and kindness. They brought themselves into the present with trips to the movies, massages and simple treats like naps answering their need for nurturing. Through consistent self-care, they taught their frightened children within that the deprivation was over and that the Nurturing Parent within would take them over any rough spots.

Claudia

You know, I still have a hard time believing my mother created this situation intentionally. She is a very strong, very intelligent person and she always found the ideas of tying kids to your apron strings repulsive. She didn't even want to be a mother. I was "an accident," she said. But I can't deny she did everything in the book to hold on to THIS accident! I guess it doesn't matter whether she did it consciously or unconsciously. The fact is, I was wrong.

Where I thought she was strong, she was weak. Where I thought she was weak, she was strong. Once I understood — even if she didn't — there was no turning back. Understanding, I could only say *goodby*. Understanding gave me no other choice. And it gave me the strength that I never thought I'd have.

For the first time in my life, I feel like a slim woman in some other fat woman's body. I feel reborn as my own mother.

An Affirmation To Stop Compulsive Eating
And Start Healthy Living

I deserve to be happy. I release any need I may have to limit my health and happiness through eating and carrying excess fat. I look to myself, not others, for the ways I want to be. I seek new interests to keep my life stimulating and fun. Every day I am awakening to fresh capacities for peace, love and self-acceptance.

NINE

Reparenting: You Can Do A Much Better Job

The saying goes, "You've come a long way, baby," but the fact of the matter is that until we go through reparenting, we haven't gone far at all from our childhood adaptations.

The sophistication we've gained since we were kids, all the skills and experience, and our abilities developed in dealing with people, mask very well an essential truth: Our psychological condition doesn't change much throughout our adult life unless we go to work on it. Once we've buried something as children without really understanding it, it continues to haunt us for decades until we are sufficiently motivated to take it out and examine it carefully. Sometimes that takes the help of a professional if we are stuck in a narrow perspective, but it certainly can be done alone or with the help of books such as this and others on family dynamics.

Our Inner Child

There is a part of us that stays a kid forever and never grows up. It is a wonderful part of us — our playful self that's always ready for fun. This Inner Child loves, is creative, spontaneous and is uncontaminated by all the garbage that has been dumped on it from various sources.

This Inner Child also remembers. It remembers everything that happened to us — the good, the bad and the ugly, the confusing, the unresolved conflicts. As adults, we carry around the resentment, hatred, fear and anxiety — all the unfinished business of our childhood.

If, as an adult, you don't trust yourself with food, you probably learned not to trust yourself as a child. Much of this learning was handed down by an authority figure like a parent, your only source of information back then about how the world worked. Getting to know your Inner Child and learning to heal your past is an excellent place to begin in learning to trust yourself.

Predictably, there can be conflicts between your decisions as an adult and the impulses of your Inner Child. Inside a 55-year-old woman there may be a 10-year-old girl who is eating to get even with Mommy for rejecting her. This is a very common scenario. As adults we may want to lose weight but find ourselves rebelling against these efforts.

When you were a child you may have been nurtured with food by others or learned to use food to nurture yourself. Perhaps your parents were too busy working, drinking or fighting with each other to give you the love and care that you needed. Food may have been a way for you to ease the pain and fear. Today, your Inner Child still craves food when nurturing is needed — the old, unresolved way, providing the self-care and nurturance you missed as a child. Formerly, your Inner Child didn't have an adult like you to help find a better way. Now it does.

The Inner Parent

Transactional Analysis is the therapeutic method that gave us the concepts of parent, adult and child ego states (see Fig. 3). The Inner Parent consists of both a Nurturing Parent and a Critical Parent. Most compulsive eaters have a very well developed Critical Parent. If your Critical Parent predominates, you may use the tactic of hating yourself into submission. You may entertain an underlying belief that the self-criticism is helping. Sounds like an idea a parent would endorse? Quite so, but few pounds have been lost through self-hatred and NO pounds at all have been kept off by this method. The myth that criticism works probably comes from those self-effacing people with critical parents who succeeded in spite of, not because of, harassment.

There has to be another way, and there is.

The parenting part of yourself feels and behaves the way that your mother and father felt and behaved. There are many parental injunctions still lurking in our conscious and unconscious mind. Have you ever heard yourself saying something exactly the way your mom or dad did? Your next thought is "Oh, my gosh, I sound just like Mom or Dad." And that's usually not meant as a compliment. This phenomenon is very common. It's as though we as children had been tape-recording everything that our parents said and felt. As adults we find ourselves running this tape of what we learned. This is the Inner Parent.

If you have children of your own, you have certainly seen this effect in your parenting behavior. You find yourself nurturing, criticizing, loving and disciplining in many of the same ways your parents did with you.

The Critical Parent

Let's hear some of this parent's favorite sayings regarding weight:

"You shouldn't have eaten that . . . you'll never be able to lose the weight."

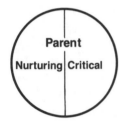

Parent — Adult — Child

When you are in the Parent ego state you feel and behave the same way your mother/father did.
Can be critical or nurturing or both. Slogans that characterize the:

Nurturing Parent

"You can do it."
"I accept you as you are."
"Even though you ate that, I love you anyway."

Critical Parent

"You shouldn't have eaten that. You are bad."
"You'll never lose weight."
"You are weak and a failure."

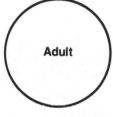

The Adult is the part of yourself that figures things out and uses facts to make decisions. Says things like: "You're overweight, it's time to cut back on intake."
"These are the proper foods to eat."

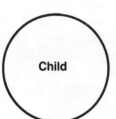

The Child part of you is what you were when you were little. She/he has the same feelings and the same ways of behaving you had when you were young.
Says things like: "I want what I want when I want it."
"That tastes good and I'm going to eat it all."
"I feel like eating."

Example: A woman who had just eaten a whole bag of cookies said:

"I knew exactly what I was doing."
    Adult
"I shouldn't have done it."
    Critical Parent
"But I felt like doing it anyhow."
    Child

Figure 3. Ego States

Learn to tell which part of you is in control.

1. Look at your behavior when you are eating compulsively.

2. How are you sitting?
   Are you huddled in a ball in a chair acting like a child who's sneaking something and afraid to get caught?
   Are you driving around eating as fast as you can so your family doesn't know what you've been doing?

3. If the answer is *yes,* then you are in your child ego state while you are eating compulsively.

4. All three ego states are important but you should have all three parts in balance. Otherwise, if you stay stuck in the:
   Child Ego state you can't stop eating.
   Parent Ego state you can never enjoy the pleasure of eating.
   Adult Ego state you would probably be extremely healthy but very boring and have no spice in life.

"You're too fat."

"You have no right to get as angry as that."

"You're imagining things."

"It wasn't that big of a deal."

"You should be able to do it. You shouldn't tell them *no*."

"You should feel guilty."

Sad, isn't it? So many of the people I've talked to continually abuse themselves with these ancient scoldings in the belief that if their parents used them, they must be helpful. I asked one particular client to give me a running commentary of messages from her Critical Parent. After doing this exercise, she said, "I never realized how critical I am of myself!" Following is the dialogue that she reported as coming from her critical parents at various times:

"You're fat."

"Your hair is frizzy."

"Your complexion isn't clear."

"You're an insecure wimp."

"You know this stuff, you never put it to use."

"You're old, out of shape and unhealthy."

"You're not professional or sophisticated enough."

"You're not intuitive enough."

"You're not focused enough."

And there was more. She called herself boring, very judgmental, too aloof, too distant, cold, hateful and mean, stupid, not responsive. She said, "You don't express yourself clearly" and, last but not least, "Your house isn't clean enough."

Hard to believe that all this was coming from a gentle, friendly and open woman who just ate too much. Make your own inventory of criticisms and see how derivative they sound. Aren't most of them echos from childhood and a de-humanizing ideal of perfection?

The Nurturing Parent

The Nurturing Parent is the side of you that is encouraging, supportive and loving. For many of us, this is but a small voice in an ocean of recrimination. It is the side from which we talk to a friend with problems but seldom to ourselves.

People who lose weight permanently, dropping the habit of cyclical compulsive eating, do it through becoming their own best friend. They support a strong Nurturing Parent. By strengthening your Nurturing Parent you can learn to support yourself through the process of becoming healthy. Without self-nurturance, self-criticism automatically takes over. In other words, if the Nurturing Parent is not strong and active, the Critical Parent will swing into action. When this happens, it leads to hopelessness and despair.

Here are some examples of messages from the Nurturing Parent:

"You're good."

"You're loving."

"You're okay just the way you are."

"It's okay, you don't have to be perfect."

"You deserve to be happy."

"You deserve to have time to yourself."

"Your body is beautiful and acceptable right now."

"You can do it."

"All isn't lost; I'll help you get it together again."

The Adult

The Adult ego state is the part of you that figures things out by simply looking at the facts. Your thoughts are, "I'm 50 pounds overweight and it's uncomfortable. I will do something about this." There's no emotion in that, just fact. That kind of information comes from your Adult self. As a healthy Adult you seek out information upon which to base your decisions. You say to yourself, "I need to know what the correct foods to eat are — which are most nutritious and what they represent in terms of calories." When you hear yourself making a statement like this, you are listening to your Adult taking charge. The Adult part of you simply observes facts, gathers information and makes decisions.

Conclusions that come from this Adult decision-making process may include thoughts such as, "My body is in poor condition, so I must exercise." The information is very clear and straightforward. You will not hear confusing messages. The Adult self does not use words like *should* and *ought*. The only information that the Adult provides is direct and to the point. When your Nurturing Parent and Child are in harmony, the Adult is free to take charge and act in your best interest. The greater your love and acceptance of yourself, the stronger you are as an Adult.

Reparenting Yourself: The Process

Visualize yourself as a kind, Nurturing Parent. This is the same person you show to those in your life who receive your love.

Take that person who has been turned outward toward the world and practice turning this self inward toward you.

Now visualize your Inner Child. See yourself at an age before you could have done anything you would consider intentionally very wrong. This may be at the age of two or three years, or even infancy.

When you overeat, draw upon that loving, compassionate parent within who sees beyond the great mountain of impressions and experience you've accumulated to the value of the little child. This greater, parenting self knows that you've been punished enough with pounds. Guilt and shame are not necessary and are inappropriate. Your nurturing Inner Parent knows that the uncomfortable feelings will be enough to let you know when you have overeaten.

This wise, parenting self also knows that even though the little kid got into the cabinet and ate all the candy bars, this child still needs and deserves love.

Love does not discriminate between chubby or fat. The parenting part of you can recognize what is happening and say, "Oh, there is fat collecting again on my body. Where did I get off track? What are the needs that I have been overlooking? I need to pay closer attention to you, my Inner Child. I want to feed you with love, not excess food. Excess food makes you feel heavy and bad. I love you too much to do that to you."

Through the reparenting process, you gently guide yourself into more health, peace and contentment. When you feel whole, there is no empty space to fill. You experience yourself as complete; the adult part of you is empowered to take charge, help you make healthful life choices. You also begin to make energy-enhancing choices with food. Through the parenting skills that you learned from your mom and dad, you have been taking care of your Inner Child through misguided nurturance.

This is what compulsive eating is about. You just have not known other ways of caring for yourself. Your Critical Parent has been engaged in the only effort it knows to get matters under control. It has been trying to help you through punishment. Most people were raised with punishment as the primary form of establishing control. It is natural, then, that under these circumstances this is what your internal Critical Parent is going to engage in when it sees that you are out of control.

You are now free to release the old, ineffective forms of parenting you picked up as a child. Through practicing the skills described in this book, you can create a strong and nurturing Inner Parent. This enables you to give love to your Inner Child through gentle yet powerful guidance. You can replace food with love as your chosen form of nurturance. You can allow natural consequences, not criticism, to guide your behavior.

Rocking Your Inner Child

The most familiar picture we all share universally as an example of nurturing is the mother picking up a crying baby and popping a bottle into its mouth. What a strong message for the effectiveness of problem-solving with food! But there are other ways.

A reparenting exercise I personally have used and recommended through the years has had powerful results. To
perform this exercise, take a few minutes each day when
you can be alone. Pick a special place in a room with no
distractions. Sit in a chair or on the floor. You may want to
set the mood by lighting a candle and dimming the lights.

Visualize your Inner Child. Imagine holding her or
him. Touch the child's soft skin and silky hair. Feel the
warm little body in your lap. It may help to hold a pillow
or have a stuffed animal or doll which can represent your
Inner Child.

Close your eyes and hold the child closely. Begin to rock
gently and talk to her or him. Say soothing words like, "I
love you, baby, just the way you are. The suffering is over.
I am with you, now. You are special to me. Your needs are
important. I am glad you are a part of me."

As you speak these loving, kind words to your Inner
Child, you begin to feel the words within yourself. The
more you do this visual action exercise, the more vivid it
will become. As you speak to the child, let the compassionate, loving parent part of you completely calm and
soothe your child self. You will experience a wonderful
feeling of well-being.

Let yourself bask in this peace as all tensions and worries leave your mind and body. Continue this for 10-20
minutes. When you finish this exercise, imagine bringing
your Inner Child into your body where it will reside as you
go through your day. For many people, the Inner Child
resides in the heart or stomach area. Throughout the day,
if you notice this child self calling out to you because it is
tired, feels frustrated or neglected or needs love, you can
reach up and touch the area where it resides. Say to it, "I
hear you. You are important and I am listening."

In the past, when you heard this inner voice calling you,
you probably fed it because this is how most of us were
taught to love. Now you are learning a new way of nurturing yourself.

Repeat this exercise several times a week. As you call
up the image of your Inner Child, you may find it appear-

ing to you at different ages. These images may represent you at different times when, as a child, you needed love or support and there was no one there to provide it.

See yourself picking up the child and saying gently, "It's okay, I'm here."

Hold and rock your child self until all the feelings of sadness or loneliness are soothed. At this time in your life you now have the power to transform your child self into a light-filled, happy youngster. It's all in your reparenting. In this way, you can heal yourself from any unresolved childhood pains. You can emotionally release your parents and take over their role. Once you really accept your Inner Child and its need for love, it becomes easier to orient your life in a self-nurturing way.

Instead of feeling selfish when you think of your child self, you will realize you are being neglectful if you don't. Your Inner Child is you and, as you've seen and experienced, ignoring it can only create problems for you and those you relate to.

A Dialogue With An Inner Child

Gail, a woman I know who has made major strides through intensive therapy, was in the process of reparenting her Inner Child when she wrote the following poem. (The *NP is Nurturing Inner* Parent, the *IC*, Inner Child.)

With Little Gail At Riverside Park

NP: Little Gail, here we are at Riverside Park!

IC: Let's play! Okay? Let's go walking on the rocks at the water's edge!

NP: Do you like to walk on the rocks near the water and look for shells and other things?

IC: Look! Come and see what I've found.

NP: There is beauty here for us to share. You and I. A piece of driftwood hollowed out. Insects and worms and water have shaped it so.

IC: Can we keep it? Can we?

NP: You have found a treasure? I'm not sure we can keep it

but I'll ask. You certainly found a treasure, hollowed out, as open as you are. As open as I am becoming.

IC: Let's keep it! Okay?

NP: You found a treasure — a simple piece of driftwood — which will be forevermore a symbol of my openness. You found a treasure — open, as you are. It will be precious and so deeply loved by me.

IC: Oh, good! I'm glad we're going to keep it. Can we take it home now?

When Gail came back from one of her follow-up sessions, she reported a tremendous reduction in food intake as a result of these dialoguing exercises. She was able to leave food on her plate and had already lost weight. She had a twinkle in her eye and a lightness to her step. The depression had lifted from her entire system and she was revitalized with life. You can give yourself this same wonderful gift of your own love.

More Mirror Talk

Another powerful Inner Child exercise is Mirror Talk. Take time when you are alone to sit in front of a mirror. Look deeply into your eyes and talk to yourself. If you look deep enough, you will see the child inside. Whenever you feel afraid, worried or sad, you can use this technique to soothe yourself.

As you look into your eyes, allow your wise, compassionate parenting self to emerge. Talk to the reflection of the person you see in the mirror, and tell this mirror self that it's okay, not to worry. You will see the fear in your eyes lessening. A calm will come over your face. You will be surprised at how much power you have to soothe, nurture and love yourself.

Rubber Ducky Therapy

Do little things for your Inner Child, like taking bubble baths. Invite a rubber ducky to play with you, if you've always wanted one. Water has amazing healing qualities. You know this to be true if you've ever sunk down into a warm bath and felt your body yielding to the healing liquid. Allow yourself a soothing bath daily.

Knead Your Needs

Massage also can be a wonderful way of nurturing your Inner Child. We are very tactile beings. Children get touched all the time but as adults, we seldom get our quota. Allow yourself the luxury of receiving and being soothed by a healing massage. Massage also can help you claim your body and feel great in it. There are many delightful things you can do to reparent and nurture your Inner Child.

More Nurturings

Get in the habit of talking to your Inner Child daily. Look at your clothes. Have you been putting the same old clothes on for months? When is the last time you did anything new for your child self? Go shopping and let the kid in you explore. Buy fun clothes (see Fig. 4). Schedule time with fun friends who are upbeat. Avoid those who burden your Inner Child with bad feelings. When you schedule your day and make commitments, ask yourself, "Am I overburdening my Inner Child? Is this too much for it?" Treat this person that you are inside with as much care and consideration as you would your child by birth. The Inner Child is no less significant.

When loving guidance is provided, you give that precious child within permission to be and to have needs. You then start the process of seeking out other new ways of feeling good. You begin the process of opening up to the world, loving life and eating to live, not living to eat (see Fig. 5).

It's important to reward yourself so your Inner Child feels loved, safe and secure inside.

Make a list of 5 things you would like to receive other than food.

1. _____

2. _____

3. _____

4. _____

5. _____

Give yourself one of these things every time you choose healthier options for yourself.

Figure 4. Rewarding Yourself For Success

Gail Writes A Poem To Her Child Within

It's true! I have neglected you
    for so long a time!
I have made myself too busy
    to be aware of how you feel.
I have not listened when you
    spoke to me or cried.
(Many times I didn't even hear.)
So, I have grimly stuffed you full
    and crammed you down inside.
But now! Now, I realize just how
    remiss I have been!
I CONSCIOUSLY
Open my heart; I pick you up;
I bring you here within.
Now, within my breast, you may live, you may
    run, you may laugh and you may play!
When you want me to, I will hold you;
    I'll listen carefully to what you say.
I will hold you very closely when you
    need to be reassured.
My hands hold no threat! My touch
    is soothing — a balm healing all your hurts.
Feel my love! My precious Child! I know now we
    are one. In loving you, I am filled.

Compulsive eating often results from the Inner Child having feelings that the Parent doesn't know how to help. The Child Ego state takes over for a time and the binge occurs. In an effort to regain control, the Critical Parent kicks in and the end result is misery. To break the pattern, use the New Way illustrated below.

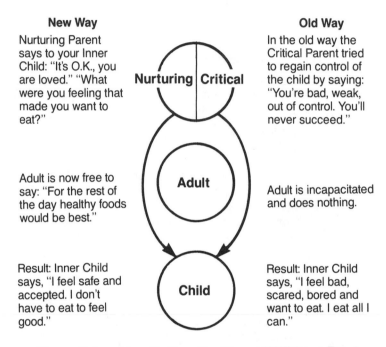

New Way

Nurturing Parent says to your Inner Child: "It's O.K., you are loved." "What were you feeling that made you want to eat?"

Adult is now free to say: "For the rest of the day healthy foods would be best."

Result: Inner Child says, "I feel safe and accepted. I don't have to eat to feel good."

Old Way

In the old way the Critical Parent tried to regain control of the child by saying: "You're bad, weak, out of control. You'll never succeed."

Adult is incapacitated and does nothing.

Result: Inner Child says, "I feel bad, scared, bored and want to eat. I eat all I can."

Figure 5. Learning To Care For Yourself Without Food
(continued)

One step further in this process is to utilize your Nurturing Parent to help yourself find new ways of comforting your Inner Child before the eating occurs.

Old Way

Inner Child feels angry or hurt and says: "I'm mad at so-and-so, I want a doughnut."

New Way

Nurturing Parent says to Inner Child: "You have a right to feel angry. Let's go talk to him/her about it. We'll find a solution."

Adult is now able to take action effectively.

Inner Child then feels the relief of being acknowledged and doesn't need to eat to feel better.

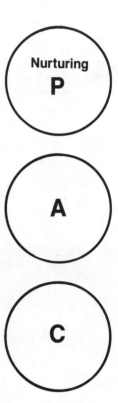

Figure 5. (Continued from previous page)

An Affirmation To Stop Compulsive Eating
And Start Healthy Living

I thoroughly enjoy taking care of myself. I nourish and nurture my body with loving attention. With every breath, I breathe in more life, joy and happiness. I like who I am as a person. I respond to all aspects of myself. I like taking charge of my life and my behavior patterns. I am the master of my life and I make it what I want it to be.

TEN

Breaking The Compulsive Eating Cycle

It may shock us whenever we find that a problem we thought was very personal actually is shared by millions of people and has been written about and dissected by professionals so often that we wonder how we can justify a tear shed on our behalf.

Nevertheless, we do deserve compassion. "Knowledge is power," said a famous compulsive eater, George Washington, but knowledge is just Part One. We have to be able to weather the process of internalizing it — that is, replacing automatic, programmed responses to situations with healthy, aware action springing from real understanding. That takes time. It means patience and a little suffering around the edges as we relapse, acknowledge our humanness and gently return to the most important task at hand. Because by now you may have gathered that what breaking the compulsive eating cycle is about is not simply wanting fewer cookies but demanding our share of the good life.

Permanent weight loss comes only with improved self-regard. Plunge wholeheartedly and holistically into learning about yourself!

The Notorious Nine Flags

Now, equipped with the psychological and practical equipment to get off the not-so-merry-go-round of compulsive eating, we can concentrate on increasing our awareness. Whenever we get caught up in the compulsive eating cycle (see Fig. 6 and Chart 3), we will recognize very vividly each of the nine stages of the cycle. Mark them with red flags and if you're not quite ready to drop any of them, still pause for a moment to allow your new understanding a chance to jump in and erode a bit more of the old programming.

Stepping Off The Cycle

No. 1 - The Feeling Point

Boredom, sadness, anger — these are the primary triggers of a compulsive eating episode. When you feel them coming on, you can now make a conscious choice whether to temporarily resolve them with food or to experiment with the alternatives we've discussed in this book.

You no longer stifle anger but talk it out compassionately. Decide what you want to say, set up a time, if necessary, to talk, and explain your position with statements emphasizing *I feel this*, not *You're bad because. . .* In this way you have increased opportunity for a positive outcome. You may not always be able to change the situation entirely but you have confirmed the importance of your feelings. This is essential in building self-esteem and overcoming compulsive behaviors.

Dwelling on sadness is clinging to the past because you haven't called on your Nurturing Parent to comfort that Inner Child. Be ready with other outlets for its emotional nature. This "pre-need" approach is essential to overcom-

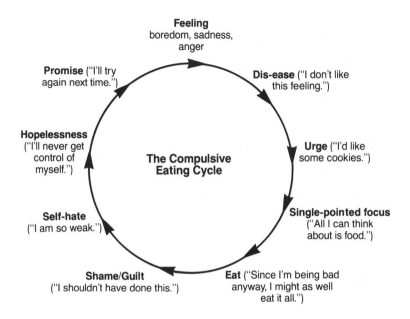

Figure 6. The Compulsive Eating Cycle

Chart 3.

Breaking The Compulsive Eating Cycle

1. You can break the Compulsive Eating Cycle at any point and if done consistently it can help you adapt new behaviors.

   Example: After compulsive eating, instead of hating and criticizing yourself, affirm and nurture yourself. Give yourself support and ask yourself what triggered it. Listen to your body.

   Note: Geneen Ruth's book, *Feeding the Hungry Heart and Breaking Free From Compulsive Eating* can help you in this process.

2. Stop the deprivation by allowing yourself to have what you want.

3. Trust yourself.

4. Listen to yourself and your body and what it's telling you, i.e.
   > I've had enough . . .
   > I need alone time . . .
   > I want to say no . . .

5. Pay attention to what you are feeling before you start eating or while you are eating.

   Example: boredom, anger, fear

6. Use the resolution format or the Breaking the Anger Trap to take new action instead of eating.

ing boredom attacks, also. Line up alternate resources before you need them instead of frantically trying to find fulfillment at the last minute.

No. 2 - The Dis-Ease Point

A follow-up to the previous condition. Boredom, sadness and anger are very uncomfortable feelings. Usually they feel as though they're going to last forever unless we eat them away.

No. 3 - The Urge Point

"I'm hungry." To break the cycle at The Urge Point, practice Thought Stopping before your urge turns into an obsession. Immediately stop yourself and say, "No, that food won't feel good to my body" or a similar statement that represents what you usually feel afterwards. This rational thought wouldn't have held up before you began understanding compulsive eating in depth but now it triggers recall of the new realities you're beginning to make a part of yourself.

No. 4 - The Single-Pointed Focus

"Nothing is going to stand between me and the refrigerator." All right, acknowledge that deprivation won't work. But walk very slowly instead of rapid-walking to the fridge. Give yourself time for your new sense of your past and yourself to assert. Don't worry if it doesn't halt the march at first. It takes practice.

No. 5 - The Eating Point

When you really want to stop a compulsive eating episode which may be headed toward a full-blown binge, remember that you are in control. Dare yourself to destroy the unnecessary food during a moment when you're feeling strong. In other words, trash the trash. Running water over it and soaking it thoroughly will prevent you from getting it out of the garbage and eating it, if you are ever so inclined. And watch how you feel immediately afterwards. You may be amazed at how fast the sense of loss drops away and is replaced by a sense of relief and empowerment. That will happen only if you have not neglected discovery work and other self-care practices we've been discussing.

Another way to deal with this stage is to watch yourself eat in front of a mirror. Reflective Eating involves watching yourself taking every bite. You'll be surprised how the act of simply acknowledging to yourself what you're doing will slow you down. It prevents you from denying the reality of your behavior. In addition, you can look into your eyes during this process and see the pain fueling the eating.

Watch what you are doing instead of thinking about what you are doing. Seeing, not thinking, is believing.

In a kind, gentle voice, talk to yourself and ask yourself what the problem is. Have compassion for the suffering being you see in the mirror. Don't judge your reflection. This exercise can prepare you for the next technique we'll mention, probably the best for intervention at the eating phase in the cycle.

Slow down and eat with dignity. Doesn't this make sense? If you're going to eat something, regardless of what it is, slow down and enjoy it! Eat with dignity and taste each bite. If you are looking in the mirror, watch yourself closely. Smell the food. Gain all the enjoyment of your senses from the experience. It's important not to hide or sneak. You are not a criminal doing anything wrong. As you chew, concentrate on the food in your mouth. Slow-chewing (which, by the way, will help you digest your food much better) helps you concentrate on the food in your mouth. Make sure you're tasting it. Ask yourself:

- Is this what I really want?
- Is it filling my needs?
- Am I satisfied?

If you are serious about losing weight permanently, you will find yourself naturally cutting back as you practice this process religiously.

No. 6 And No. 7 - The Shame/Guilt Point And The Self-Hate Point

How familiar! To break the cycle at these phases, tell yourself, "It's okay, I accept you." Self-chastisement is part of the problem, not the solution. Nurturing, not hating, yourself is what permanent weight loss is all about. Most of the problem-eating occurs once the self-hate begins and you are eating to punish yourself. **Self-love gives you the strength to stop.**

- Allow yourself to try something new.
- Do not persecute yourself if you fall back.
- Take one step at a time.

You'll find yourself doing better each day that you replace self-hate with love. When you are stressed and you find yourself going back to your original behaviors, you simply grab some compassion for yourself and say, "It's okay, I love you anyway." Wouldn't you say this to a friend?

That evening or the next day, resume your normal eating patterns when you get hungry. Nurture yourself and support yourself through the process. You are conditioning yourself to move to a completely different way of being. Eventually, there's no longer a feeling of craving. You don't need to go out and eat as much as you can hold. You have learned to encourage yourself, to act as your own friend and to create a desire to eat in a healthy manner.

No. 8 - The Hopelessness Point

This is bottoming-out time. "I'll never change! It's happened again, I couldn't control it and I never will!"

That's a logical conclusion if you do not make renewal your top priority in life. But if you've been reinforcing new knowledge about yourself daily — practicing it, not just reading it or talking about it — you will move forward, inch by inch, sometimes even by a gallop.

No. 9 - The Promise Point

This is a relative of the New Year's resolution and is just as likely to happen. "Tomorrow, I'll take control." It is inspired by sheer intolerance for that hopeless feeling — and not much more.

How do you get back on the horse when you've failed for what may well be the thousandth time? It's not easy. You're down on yourself and it seems your body is working against you. If you've been eating a lot of junk food, be aware that your physiological cravings will be very high. This has nothing to do with your emotions. You also feel tired, sluggish, sleepy and perhaps stiff.

Fatigue is one of the most commonly reported reasons why people eat compulsively.

The more sensitive you become to your body, the more you recognize food overdoses and their direct effect on your body. The food is making your body feel sluggish and you are drawn to the foods that you believe will make you feel better and more energetic. When you're caught in this dilemma, you must have patience with yourself. The best cure for this syndrome is time between episodes. Give yourself a few hours before eating again or wait to eat until the next morning. Then you will feel that you can start over. Indeed, you can.

You must gently guide yourself back to healthful eating. When you have cravings for sweets, drink juice or something else that will meet your needs without the accompanying heaviness that sugar and junk food elicit.

Giving yourself permission, time and again, to start over. Even those who do not struggle with weight or dieting sometimes eat compulsively or overeat. However, there is one difference between them and you, if you have been a compulsive eater. Individuals who naturally regulate their systems will notice the discomfort in their bodies and will stop eating heavy foods until their bodies feel comfortable again. Compulsive eaters sometimes feel so much self-hate and hopelessness that they eat more because they feel so bad. Compulsive eaters often eat to punish themselves.

Leonard's One-Minute Diet

Leonard Hollander, a colleague of mine, told me that one sure-fire way of breaking the compulsive eating cycle at the Promise Point was simply to take one minute every day to stand in front of a full-length mirror, nude.

"Oh, I know well enough what I look like," you may say. So often, however, we intellectualize our mirror-image if we don't face it full-length. In our minds we modify it in various ways so that it isn't quite as difficult to face. But, in the spirit of experimentation, let's see where this exercise might lead.

First, face the mirror and see how you look. Note excess fat. Turn sideways and let your stomach relax and do what I call "checking the sidewalls." This quick method will prevent any denial you might have had about the food you've been ingesting. In a glance you will know if you've overeaten that day.

Another technique is to do stretching exercises or yoga in front of your full-length mirror. (Using this technique, I lost 30 pounds.)

Many people do not realize that there are gentle, soothing exercises that can be done at home which can have a profound effect on the body. Some believe that if they don't do aerobic exercise, there is no use in doing anything. This stems from the belief that the heart rate has to be at a certain point for exercise to be of any use. This is simply not true. All movement is good. Doing gentle stretching and moving exercises in front of a mirror can help you to quit compulsive eating in several ways.

First, you get direct feedback on eating habits. You don't
have to put on 10 or 20 pounds before you notice what is
happening. I am convinced that people whose weight fluc-
tuates this much are frequently in a state of denial. When
you begin to notice how two-pound fluctuations affect
your stomach, then you can make the necessary changes
in your eating habits.

The second way these exercises can work for you is by
relieving stress. Compulsive eating is, for many, a means
of reducing stress. When you are reducing stress in more
healthful ways, you automatically feel good about yourself. This helps to motivate you to take better care of
yourself in all ways.

**Exercise in any form is incompatible with excessive
appetite and increases your metabolism.**

A technique I used for years to help me stop compulsive
eating episodes was the one I mentioned earlier of doing
Mirror Yoga. It invalidated what had become my version
of reality. The fullness in my stomach made me feel as
though I was a walking blimp and this inevitably led to a
downward spiral of more eating and depression. Through
the process of observing myself as I stretched, I realized
that all was not lost. I, indeed, was not a blimp. There was
still hope. This realization reduced my appetite so I
stopped eating compulsively and felt motivated.

By befriending your body and acknowledging subtle
physical changes, you will be motivated to control your
eating. It doesn't take long before you notice yourself looking slimmer. Your skin will regain its tightness and you
will feel more agile and alive. This in itself helps to keep
you from compulsive eating.

**Can you develop higher priorities than food? Chal-
lenge yourself!**

Behavior-Chain Building

A behavior chain is any series of activities which you
perform in a sequence over an extended period of time.

One behavior always leads to the next. Getting up in the morning can lead to overeating that afternoon if you follow the same routines day after day. It is very hard to break a behavior chain once it has been established. That's why you must be patient with yourself. When you get into a groove, it takes repeated effort to establish a new way of behaving. Both body and mind resist it at first. It doesn't matter where you break the chain for new behavior to develop. It only matters that you do break it.

Interestingly, you don't even have to break the behavior chain at the point where you're eating to affect your eating. Try breaking it at any point. This evenually, with your other support work, will lead to breaking the entire compulsive-eating pattern.

Overeating is painful and feels bad. When you are filled with self-love, your tolerance for behaviors that create bad feelings is greatly diminished.

The Spiraling

Recovering from compulsive eating appears to be a spiraling process. You start out with heavy eating. As you progress and grow and learn to befriend your body, you begin eating less. There may be times when you feel like you've kicked the habit, and then you'll notice by the feeling in your body that you just overate.

Stressful times may also arise, causing a bout of eating. When you slip, it's hard not to become discouraged and start catastrophizing. You may tell yourself you haven't changed a bit and get into a self-hate cycle. What you need to focus on is that the time between your compulsive eating episodes is expanding.

Also notice that the quantity of food you are consuming is reducing. A year ago, an episode may have consisted of half a gallon of ice cream. Today, it may be two scoops.

You become more body-sensitive. Since the stomach in a healthy eater is only as big as a fist, it doesn't take much food for fullness to register. Previously, you probably had your stomach stretched and could eat a whole bag of chips before feeling it. Today, you eat two handfuls and feel satisfied.

Remember to stand in front of the mirror every day to see if your stomach is protruding and notice subtle changes. This will help you to cut back on your eating. You will begin to enjoy having a flat stomach and feeling light. You will tune in to your body when you want to eat. Let your body tell you when it's time to stop.

In Judy Wardell's book *Thin Within*, she outlines a simple process for weight maintenance and controlled eating based on tuning in to the body. First, she recommends that you eat only what your body really wants. You only eat at times when you are really hungry and stop eating just when you're becoming comfortable. As you empower yourself to do what's best for yourself, you can follow these guidelines and they will melt away extra weight.

Most compulsive eating is done with forbidden foods and compulsive eaters rarely give themselves what they really needed to eat. Naturally slim people eat what their bodies crave. In this way, they don't feel deprived. This lack of deprivation prevents gorging.

Befriending and listening to your body is an integral step in kicking the habit of compulsive eating and ridding yourself of excess fat. You may be surprised once you start really tuning in to your body. It will take much less food than you expect to reach that comfortably full feeling. Your body will tell you when to shelve the junk food. It will crave healthy nonfat foods. One day you will look back and realize you have spiraled through many phases of recovery. You will feel tuned in to your body and your body will guide your eating.

You eat when you're hungry and you eat what you really want.

You quit eating when you are comfortable.

You realize you are at the top of the spiral. And you feel great, inside and out!

Decisions — Past And Present

Old Decisions

In my childhood, this is how I felt:

1. The role food is supposed to play in my life is . . .
2. How I feel about my body is . . .
3. How I solve my problems or make myself feel better is through . . .
4. How I feel about myself in general is . . .

New Decisions

As an adult, here are the new decisions I want to make about myself:

1. The role I want food to play in my life is . . .
2. How I want to feel about my body is . . .
3. New ways I want to solve my problems and make myself feel better without using food are . . .
4. How I want to feel about myself is . . .

Preludes By Sara
(An excerpt)

Dream of dreams
Enlightened awakening
Prelude to new hopes of a new future
Along the horizon of life everchanging.
Misconceptions of the truth of harmony.
Each life is but an impression
Constructed on triumphs yet unknown
Of landscapes of the mind
To find the Rainbow's Source.

An Affirmation To Stop Compulsive Eating
And Start Healthy Living

I have the courage to make my life what I want it to be.

Chapter Notes

Chapter 1

Ganley, R. M., "Emotion and Eating in Obesity: A Review of the Literature." *International Journal of Eating Disorders*, v. 8-3, 343-361, 1989.

Chapter 2

Bilich, M., **Weight Loss From The Inside Out: Help For The Compulsive Eater.** San Francisco: Harper & Row, 1983.

Chapter 3

Roth, G., **Why Weight? A Guide to Ending Compulsive Eating.** New York: New American Library, 1989.

Chapter 4

LeBlanc, D., M.Ed., "Visualizations for Weight Loss." Audiocassette tape, 1988.

Pearsall, P., Ph.D., **Superimmunity: Master Your Emotions and Improve Your Health.** New York: McGraw-Hill, 1987.

Chapter 5

Jackson, I., **The Breath Play Approach to Whole Life Fitness.** New York: Doubleday, 1986.

Ponath, Suzanne, Unique Performance, Inc., P.O. Box 1178, Lake Dallas, Texas 75065.

Chapter 6

Ganley, R. M., "Emotion and Eating in Obesity: A Review of the Literature." *International Journal of Eating Disorders*, v. 8-3, 343-361, 1989.

Chapter 9

DeFoore, B., Ph.D., "Nurturing Your Inner Child." Audio-cassette tape, 1988.

Chapter 10

LeBlanc, D., M.Ed., "Compulsive Eating: You Can't Quit Until You Know What's Eating You!" 2-tape audiocassette album, 1989.

Wardell, J., **Thin Within: How To Eat And Live Like A Thin Person.** New York: Pocket Books, 1985.

Suggested Reading

Overcoming Compulsive Eating Books

Bilich, M., **Weight Loss From the Inside Out: Help for the Compulsive Eater.** San Francisco: Harper & Row, 1983.

Ganley, R.M., "Emotion and Eating in Obesity: A Review of the Literature." *International Journal of Eating Disorders*, v. 8-3, 343-361, 1989.

McFarland, B. and Baker-Baumann, T., **Shame and Body Image: Culture and the Compulsive Eater.** Deerfield Beach, FL: Health Communications.

Roth, G., **Why Weight? A Guide to Ending Compulsive Eating.** New York: New American Library, 1989.

Wardell, J., **Thin Within: How to Eat and Live Like a Thin Person.** New York: Pocket Books, 1985.

Nutrition Fitness Books

Jackson, I., *The Breath Play Approach to Whole Life Fitness*. New York, Doubleday, 1986.

Parker, V. and Gates, R., **The Lowfat Lifestyle.** LFL Associates, 52 Condolea Court, Lake Oswego, OR, 97035, 1984.

Pawlich, L., **Life Without Diets,** P.O. Box 1577, Cathedral City, CA, 92234-1577, 1989.

Pearsall, P., **Superimmunity: Master Your Emotions and Improve Your Health.** New York: McGraw-Hill, 1987.

Vartabedian, R., M.D. and Matthews, K.; **Nutripoints: The Breakthrough Point System for Optimal Nutrition.** New York: Harper & Row, 1990.

Yoga Books

Hittleman, R., **Yoga – 28 Day Exercise Plan.** New York: Bantam Books, 1988.

Welch, R., **Raquel: The Raquel Welch Total Beauty and Fitness Program.** New York: Bantam Books, 1984.

Audiocassettes

Affirmations for Weight Loss, Donna LeBlanc, M.Ed. Music by Steven Halpern, 1988. $10.50 + $2.00 S/H.

Compulsive Eating: You Can't Quit Until You Know What's Eating You! 6-tape album with workbook, Donna LeBlanc, M.Ed. Music soundtrack on tapes 9, 10, 11 and 12 by Steven Halpern, 1989. $59.95 + $3.50 S/H.

Compulsive Eating: You Can't Quit Until You Know What's Eating You! 2-tape album with workbook, Donna LeBlanc, M.Ed., 1989. $19.95 + $2.50 S/H.

Visualizations for Weight Loss, Donna LeBlanc, M.Ed. Music soundtrack by Steven Halpern, 1988. $10.50 + $2.00 S/H.

Nurturing Your Inner Child, Bill DeFoore, Ph.D. Music soundtrack by Steven Halpern, 1989. $10.50 + $2.00 S/H.

**For more information regarding tapes and the Compulsive Eating Program, contact the Institute for Personal and Professional Development, Inc., 4201 Wingren, Suite 201, Irving, Texas 75062. 800-322-4773. To order tapes, make checks payable to Personal Development Tapes, 4201 Wingren, Suite 201, Irving, Texas 75062. Texas residents, include 8% sales tax.

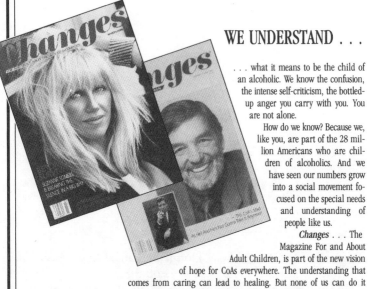